Traumatic Brain Injury - Neurobiology, Diagnosis and Treatment

Edited by Yongxia Zhou

Published in London, United Kingdom

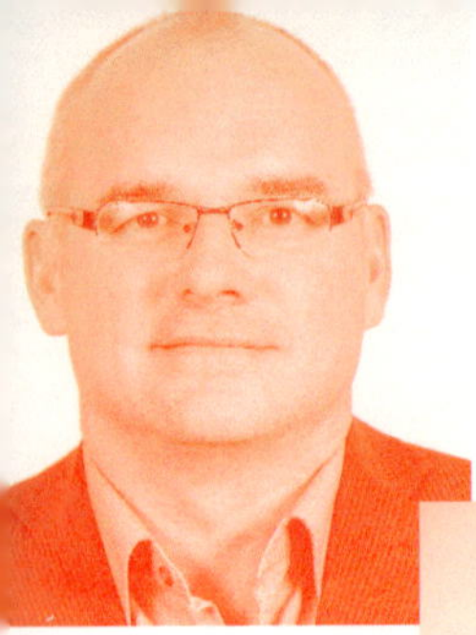
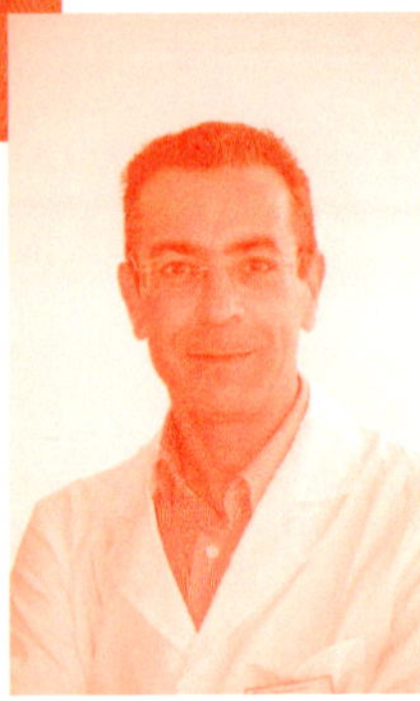
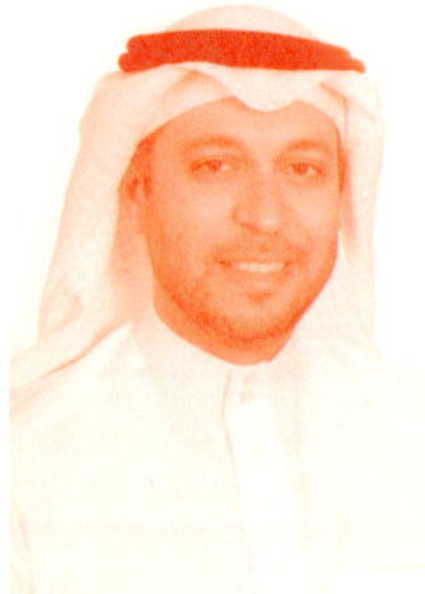
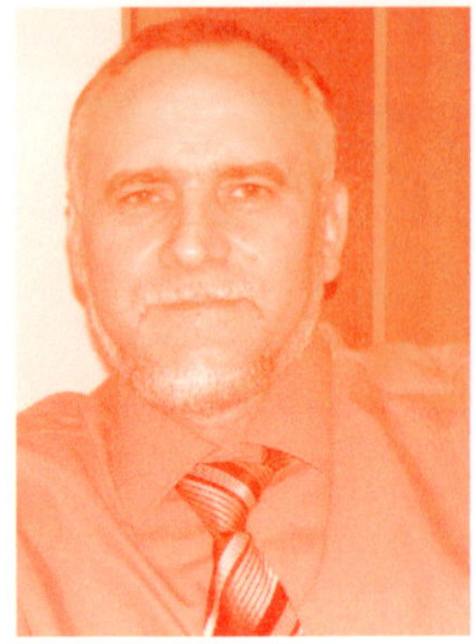
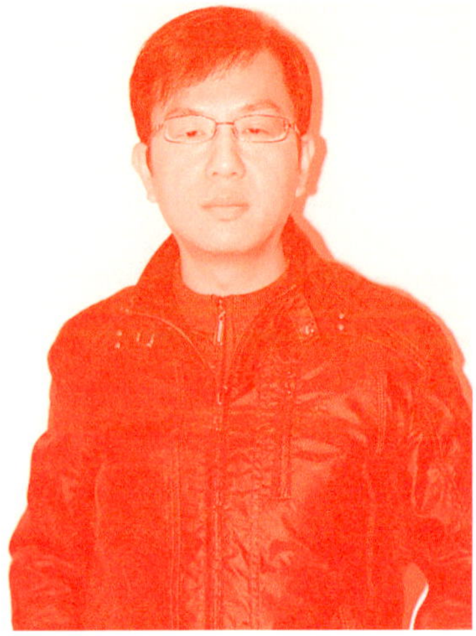
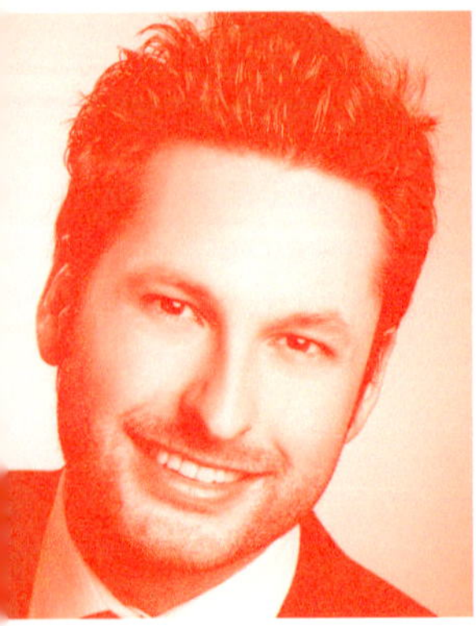
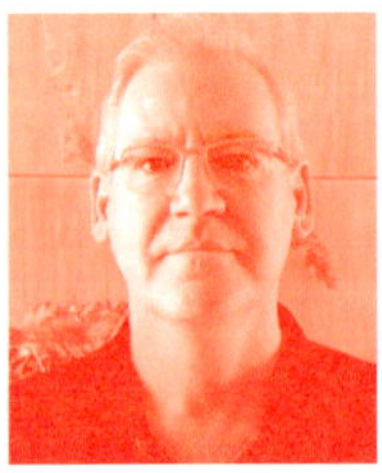

IntechOpen

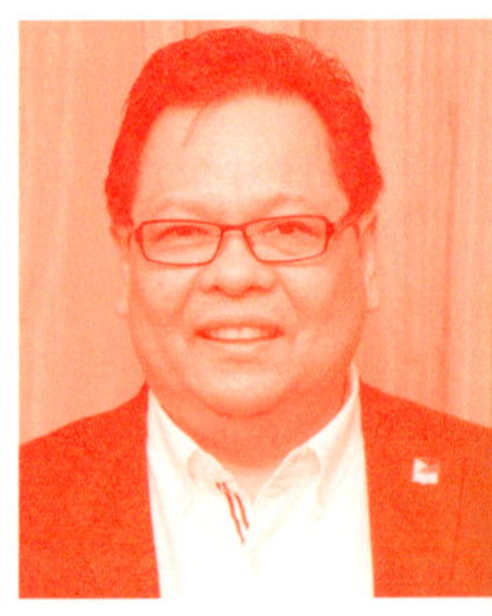
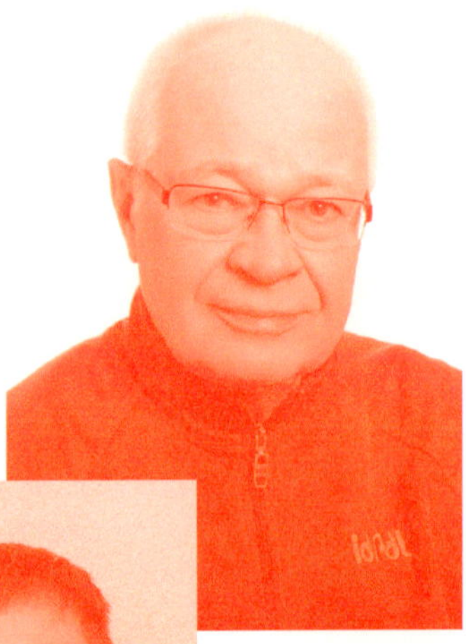
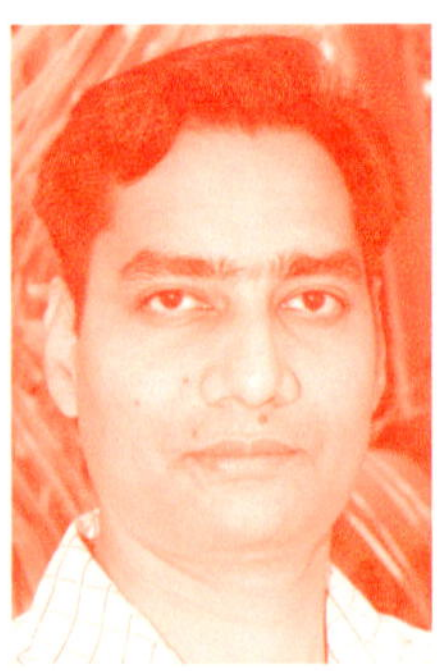
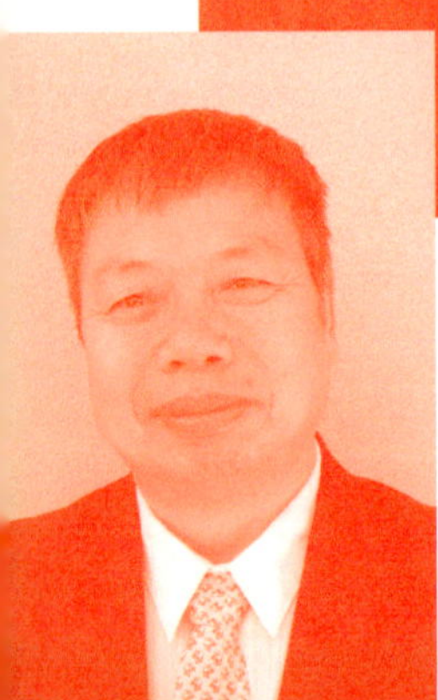
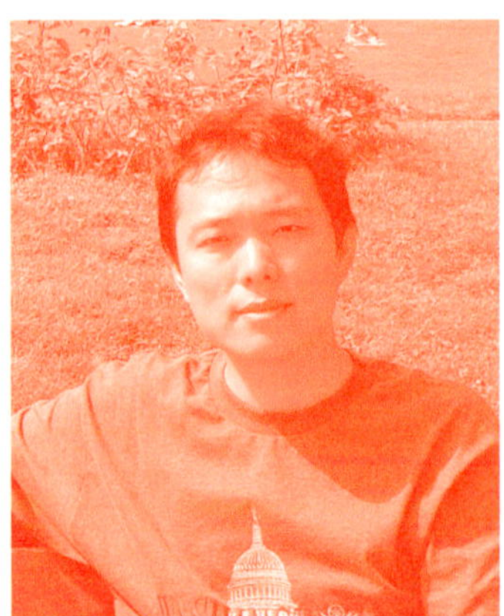
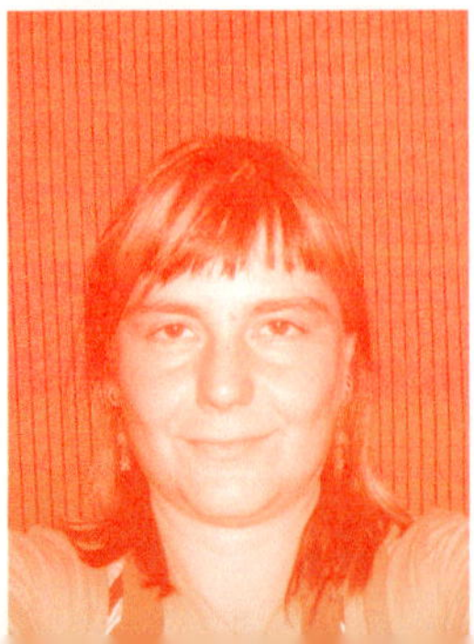

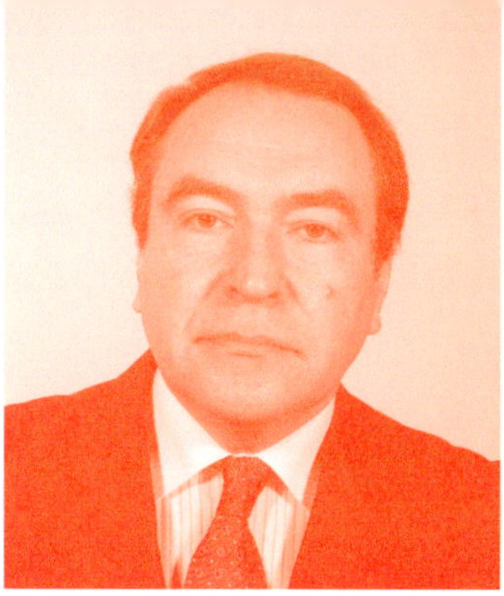
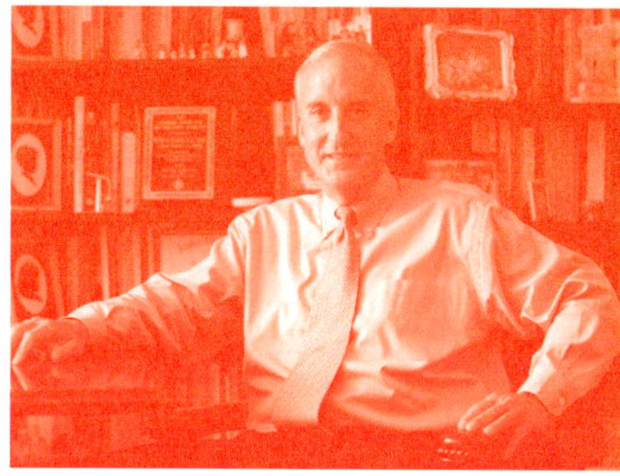
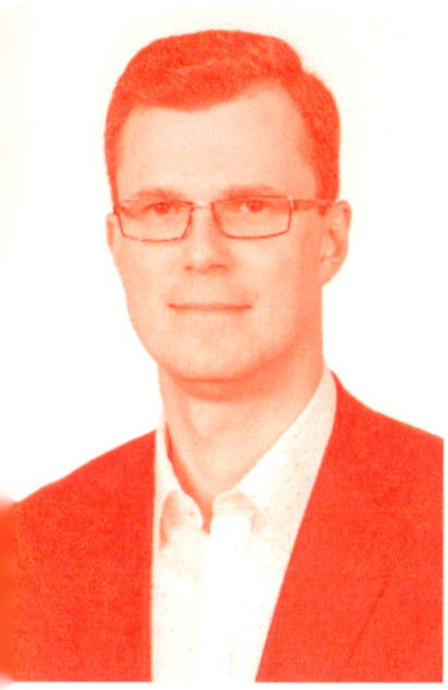
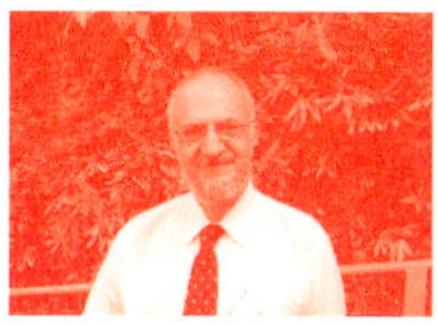
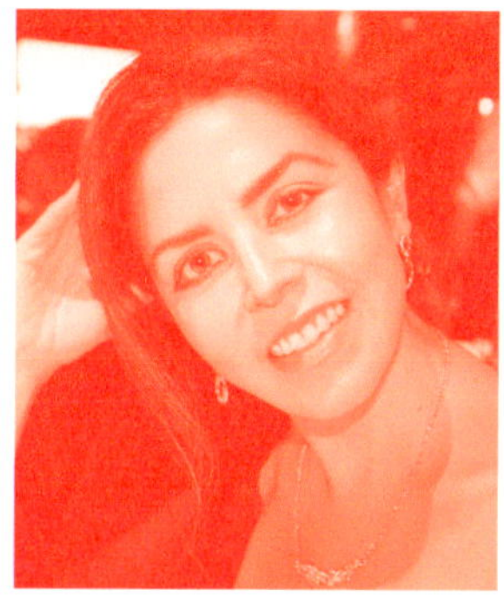

Supporting open minds since 2005

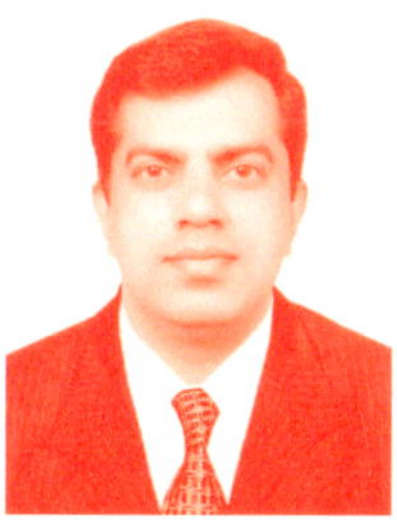
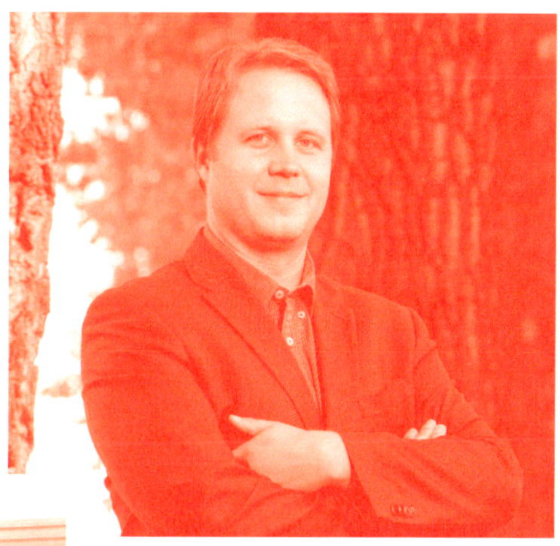
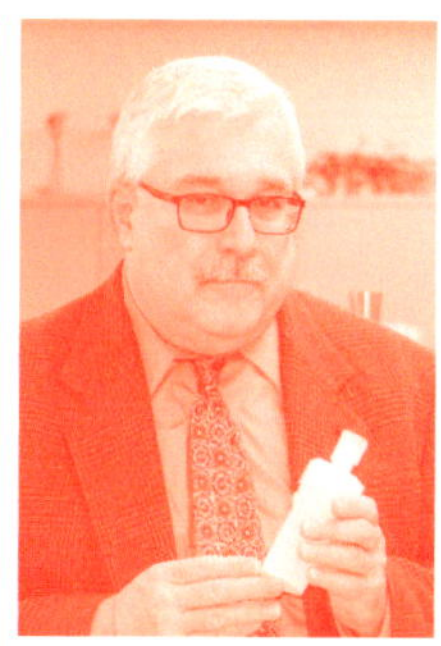
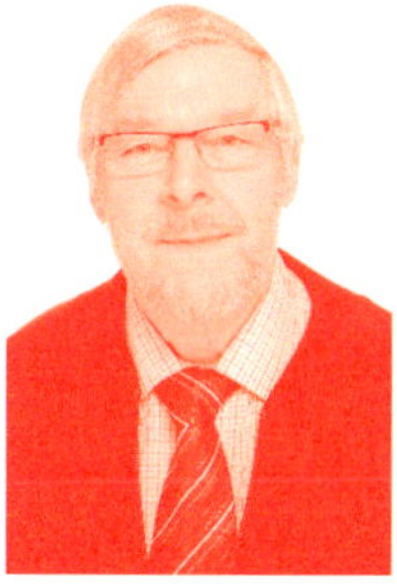
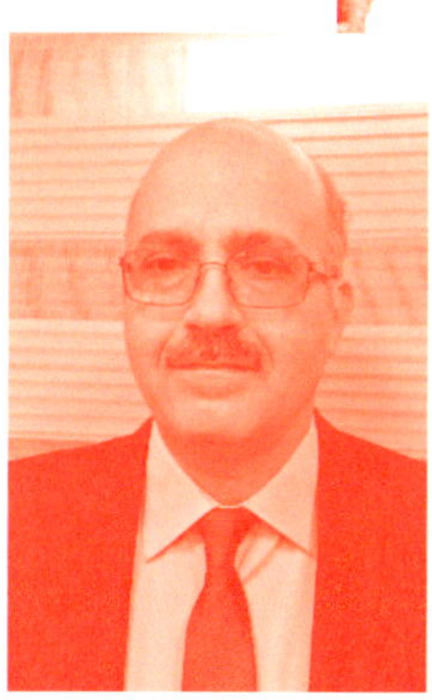
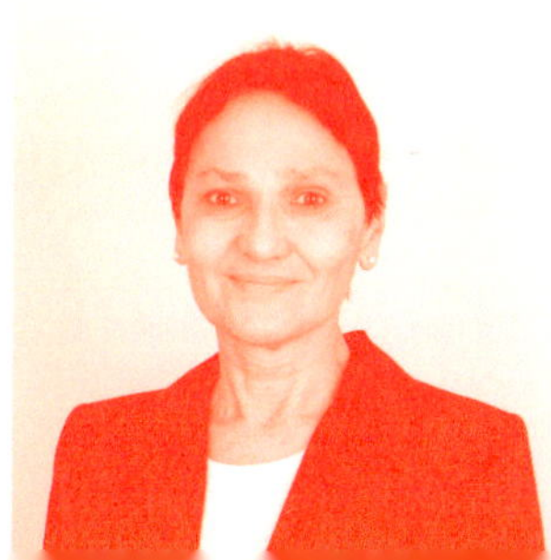
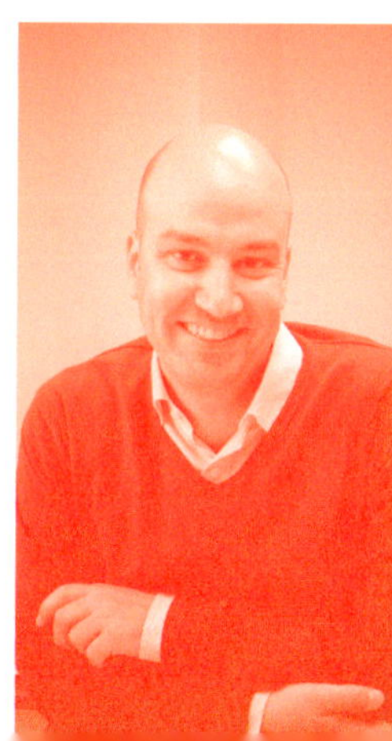

Traumatic Brain Injury - Neurobiology, Diagnosis and Treatment
http://dx.doi.org/10.5772/intechopen.77680
Edited by Yongxia Zhou

Contributors
Kathryn Nel, Saraswathie Govender, Alexander Rodríguez, Pedro Javier Villalba, Eliana Cervera, Luz Navarro, Marina Martinez-Vargas, Mercedes Graciela Porras-Villalobos, Francisco Estrada-Rojo, Ricardo Jesus Martinez-Tapia, Adan Perez-Arredondo, Antonio Barajas-Martinez, Zamzuri Idris, Ang Song Yee, Regunath Kandasamy, Asrulnizam Abd Manaf, Mohd Hasyizan Bin Hassan, Wan Nazaruddin Wan Hassan, Mohammad Nadir Nadir Haider, Itai Bezherano, Mohammad Meshkini, Ali Meshkini, Homayoun Sadeghi-Bazarghani, Rafael Badenes, Berta Monleon Lopez, Lorenzo Peluso

First published in London, United Kingdom, 2019 by IntechOpen
IntechOpen is the global imprint of INTECHOPEN LIMITED, registered in England and Wales, registration number: 11086078, The Shard, 25th floor, 32 London Bridge Street
London, SE19SG – United Kingdom
Printed in Croatia

British Library Cataloguing-in-Publication Data
A catalogue record for this book is available from the British Library

Additional hard and PDF copies can be obtained from orders@intechopen.com

Traumatic Brain Injury - Neurobiology, Diagnosis and Treatment
Edited by Yongxia Zhou
p. cm.
Print ISBN 978-1-78984-295-1
Online ISBN 978-1-78984-296-8
eBook (PDF) ISBN 978-1-78984-500-6

For EU product safety concerns:
IN TECH d.o.o., Prolaz Marije Krucifikse Kozulić 3, 51000 Rijeka, Croatia, info@intechopen.com or visit our website at intechopen.com.

Meet the editor

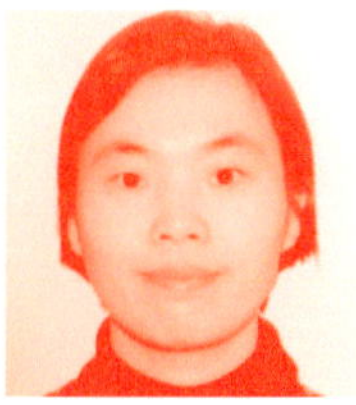

Yongxia Zhou completed her PhD from the University of Southern California in Biomedical Imaging (2004). Her research interest is radiology and neuroscience applications. She was trained and has worked as a neuroimaging scientist in several prestigious institutes, including Columbia University, University of Pennsylvania, and NIH. Her research focuses on multimodal neuroimaging integration, including MRI/PET and EEG instrumentation, and makes best use of multiple modalities to help interpret underlying disease mechanisms. She has authored more than five monograph books, and edited several books for well-known publishers, including IntechOpen and Nova Science. She has published over 100 papers and abstracts and served as a reviewer and editor for many reputed international journals and conferences.

Contents

Preface

Traumatic brain injury (TBI) is the leading cause of mortality and morbidity with a high incidence in young people all over the world. Post-concussive syndrome (PCS) is an international public health concern with 5–10% of mild TBI (mTBI) cases experiencing concussion in their lives and about 20% of patients having persistent PCS within 6 months to 1 year after mTBI. There are many advanced techniques and methods for the investigation of brain changes and treatments in TBI patients and each of these techniques provides important insights into pathophysiology due to head injury but may not be limited to conventional methods. This new information emerges to give a broad picture of TBI research and clinical evaluation such as cumulative mild head injury (CMHI), novel neuroimaging findings and biomarkers, neuroprotective treatments, brain cooling, and sedation in TBI patients, as well as neuronal and glial biomarkers.

The first section of the book introduces disease neurobiology and PCS. Chapter 1 "Post-Concussion Syndrome" describes the definition of PCS, classification, and association with brain dysfunction, blood flow regulation, intracranial pressure change, and the role of neuroinflammation, as well as long-term sequelae such as chronic traumatic encephalopathy and treatment. Discussing PCS problems in TBI for the improvement of clinical diagnosis based on several definitions is challenging given subjective and gross aspects of the assessments of PCS, e.g. Glasgow comma scale and loss of conscious. This chapter provides many characteristics of PCS, including classification, association with autonomic nervous system dysfunction, brain changes, and treatment that could serve as a reference resource for further research. Chapter 2 "Neuroprotection, Photoperiod, and Sleep" investigates the neurobiological basis of neuroprotective activation, and correlation with PCS, including sleep. The authors attempt to explain the neurobiological basis of neuroprotective activation, adaptive response to photoperiod possibly due to injury of the suprachiasmatic nucleus, and correlation with post-traumatic symptoms, including sleep, as well as limitations. This chapter provides clues to studying the relationships between neuroprotection and sleep as well as the involved neurotransmission systems.

The second section of the book covers the imaging diagnosis and biomarkers in TBI. Chapter 3 "Cumulative Mild Head Injury (CMHI) in Contact Sports" provides a CMHI review, brain changes, and risk factors. This chapter briefly overviews the structure and neuroanatomy of brain change to illustrate the pathophysiological mechanisms involved in primary and secondary head injuries. Some relatively new imaging perspectives, including diffusion axonal injury, close-head injury, homeostasis irregulation, and tauopathy, are illustrated concisely. Risk factors for all types of CMHI are described further with details for early prevention and cure. Chapter 4 "Neuronal and Glial Biomarkers Research for Traumatic Brain Injury" studies multiple biomarkers, including S-100β, UCH-L1, and GFAP for blood–brain barrier breakdown and neuronal injury. The sensitivity and specificity of each biomarker from published articles as well as the ratio between GFAP and UCH-L1 are reported with confirmative statistical results and table summaries. This chapter gives a full overview of the most promising biomarkers studied as predictors of the severity of TBI, with a special focus on their nature, location, basal concentrations, and methods by which they can be quantified efficiently in blood samples.

The third section refers to the treatment of and multiple therapeutic strategies in TBI patients. Chapter 5 "Use of Neuroprotective Agents for Traumatic Brain Injury" evaluates more than 12 neuroprotective agents from 32 studies with objective data and statistical analyses. Complete descriptions of significance, improvements, and side effects of each agent are covered in detail with the conclusion that a few agents, including oxygen, cyclosporine A, and rivastigmine use for different phases of TBI, show promising treatment effects. Authoritative statements, comprehensive citations, and confirmation with scientific and solid evidence are strong points of this chapter. Chapter 6 "Direct Brain Cooling in Treating Severe Traumatic Head Injury" addresses the interesting and promising topic of hypothermia as a neuroprotective effect in TBI patients. The benefits of cooling, especially of mild cooling such as brain oxygen level reaching desirable levels and a better Glasgow outcome scale at 6 months follow-up, are described and analyzed scientifically with a new cooling machine D-Brain therapy. This chapter highlights the encouraging results of pilot research on direct focal brain cooling therapy in severe head injury patients with significant clinical outcome results in a mild cooling group due to elevations in oxygenation level of injured and decompressed brain tissues. The last chapter "Sedation in TBI Patients" discusses sedation in TBI as a neurocritical and therapeutic strategy with different assessments. The main pharmacological principles, neurophysiology, and neuropathology of sedatives and analgesics, including propofol, benzodiazepines, and opioids, are outlined and evaluated. Several topics and properties based on new technologies, including physiological indications, status epilepticus treatment, management, monitoring in the neuro-ICU with various scales and neurologic examinations, are integrated for better diagnosis and treatment improvement.

Yongxia Zhou, PhD
Imaging Scientist,
University of Southern California and Columbia University,
Los Angeles, California, USA

Section 1

Disease Etiology and Post Concussion Syndrome

Chapter 1

Post Concussion Syndrome

Mohammad Nadir Haider and Itai Bezherano

Abstract

Post-concussion syndrome (PCS) is a complex disorder and the complete pathophysiology is still not completely understood. PCS can be subcategorized into physiological PCS, vestibulo-ocular PCS, cervicogenic PCS, and mood-related PCS based on predominant clinical signs and symptoms. Physiological PCS is the most classic type of PCS and is due to global metabolic dysfunction in the brain which affects the autonomic nervous system (ANS) and cerebral blood flow (CBF) autoregulation. This is suspected to be the cause for symptom-limited exercise intolerance which is a characteristic finding in this subtype. In this chapter we discuss the definition of PCS and the main subtypes. We further discuss possible causes for symptoms of PCS based on research that have studied this disorder using advanced imaging, cardiovascular and cerebrovascular metrics, and intracranial pressure. Finally, we discuss the treatment of PCS and the possible long-term effects.

Keywords: mild traumatic brain injury, concussion, post-concussion syndrome, autonomic nervous system dysfunction, cervical post traumatic disorder, vestibulo-ocular post traumatic disorder, exercise treatment

1. Introduction

Concussions are defined as reversible neurological dysfunction in the absence of gross brain lesions [1], caused by either a direct blow to the head, neck, or elsewhere on the body with an impulsive force transmitted to the head [2]. Although there is some ambiguity in the definitions of mild traumatic brain injury (mTBI) and concussion, the term concussion usually refers to a milder head injury (GCS = 15) and generally used in the context of sport-related injuries while mTBI are a broader term that includes concussion [3]. Concussions have become an international public health concern and it is estimated that about 42 million people suffer from some form of mTBI every year [4]. In the US alone, it is estimated that 1.6–3.8 million mTBI occur each year [5] and approximately 5–10% of the population will experience a concussion in their lives [6]. Some populations, like military personnel, are at a higher risk for concussions and mTBI. It is estimated that approximately 19.5–22.8% of all returning deployed US troops suffer exposure to blast and/or concussive TBI [7].

The pathophysiology of concussion has been studied in great detail, yet it is one of the least understood injuries facing the neuroscience or sports medicine community [8]. It is hypothesized that acceleration/deceleration and rotational forces cause diffuse injury to the neurons, which causes an ionic imbalance and release of a cascade of neurotransmitters [9–11]. To restore homeostasis, membrane pumps become activated which results in a brief hyper-metabolic state. Lactate is produced, which further impairs neuronal function [12]. Intra-axonal alterations within in the subaxolemmal, neurofilament, and microtubular cytoskeleton network with impairment of axonal transport as well as impaired glucose metabolism have been observed in the acute and subacute phase after mTBI, which support the hypothesis of metabolic and cellular disruptions in the brain [13].

The typical duration of clinical recovery in majority of concussions is 7–10 days, but it is estimated that 10% [14] to 30% [15] of adolescents and 10–15% [16, 17] of adults take much longer to recover. These statistics have ranged from 5% to more than 50% in the published literature; the primary cause of this variation is due to the different criteria used to measure dysfunction [18]. If symptoms persist for more than 2 weeks in adults, or 1 month in adolescents, then the diagnosis of post-concussion syndrome (PCS) is made [19]. However, this terminology is incorrect because technically it is not a *syndrome*. A *syndrome* is a consistent set of findings associated with a condition with symptom linkage and of symptom resolution [20], but currently there is no gold-standard symptom or set of symptoms that are diagnostic of PCS [21] or its recovery [22]. PCS is defined in the World Health Organization's International Classification of Disease 10 (ICD-10) as history of head trauma with or without loss of consciousness preceding at least three of the following symptoms: headache, dizziness, malaise, fatigue, noise tolerance; irritability, depression, anxiety, emotional lability; subjective concentration, memory, or intellectual difficulties without neuropsychological evidence of marked impairment; insomnia; reduced alcohol tolerance; and preoccupation with above symptoms [23].

Self-reported symptom checklist have been used to report the symptoms of a concussion, the most common being the post-concussion symptom scale (PCSS) [24]. It is a list of 22-symptoms, which can be rated on a Likert scale (no symptom to severe symptom), with a maximum possible score of 132. Unfortunately, these symptoms are not specific to concussions or PCS and the healthy population has an average score of 6 out of 132 [25], hence several studies use the cutoff of 7 on the PCSS to diagnose concussion and PCS [22]. However, there is no symptom cutoff limit that can reliably identify people with concussion and/or PCS. One study [26] showed this cutoff criterion (7 out of 132) incorrectly labeled 34% of healthy people with PCS, which is higher than people with a concussive head injury (31%). Self-reported symptom checklists have also been criticized because there is variation in symptom reporting between people. Athletes are known to under-report their symptoms, whereas people with secondary gain are known to over-report them [27]. Another potential downside of symptom checklists is that it is suggested to reinforce illness behavior and encourages over-endorsement of symptoms that might not otherwise have been reported on free recall [28, 29]. Still, this is a useful tool for clinicians because it helps track symptoms longitudinally, so it is always advised to compare symptom reports with previous ones. Another popular symptom checklist is the post-concussion symptom inventory (PCSI), it has an added benefit which allows patients to report symptoms before and after head injury which makes is easier for clinicians to interpret its findings [30].

2. Post-concussion syndrome classification

PCS have been subcategorized based on their predominant pathophysiology as shown in **Figure 1** [31, 32]. These classifications may overlap as it is possible to have one or more associated conditions after a head injury. Physiological PCS are believed to be true concussions because these patients typically present with minimal physical examination abnormalities but can have signs of oculomotor and/or vestibular dysfunction. They often complain of cognitive fatigue, headaches, and

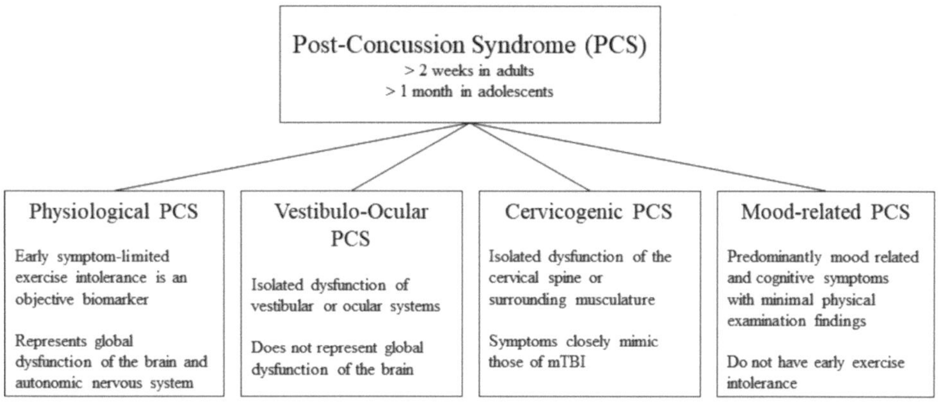

Figure 1.
Post-concussion syndrome subtypes. Classification of the different types of PCS based on predominant clinical signs and symptoms.

balance problems [33], but the most objective biomarker of physiological dysfunction is symptom-limited exercise intolerance at a low heart rate [34]. These patients have worsening of existing symptoms, or onset of new symptoms, when they begin to exercise. This exacerbation occurs at below 70% of their age appropriate maximum heart rate [32]. The pathophysiology of this type of PCS will be discussed later in more detail.

Vestibulo-ocular and cervicogenic PCS are not true concussions since they do not involve global metabolic disturbance of brain function, rather post-traumatic disorders of isolated subsystems from which the symptoms originate, i.e., the central oculomotor and vestibular systems and upper cervical spine respectively [35]. They present with predominantly vestibulo-ocular/cervical signs and symptoms, respectively, and may demonstrate exercise intolerance during graded treadmill testing, but symptom exacerbation typically occurs at a significantly greater workload (beyond 70% of age-predicted maximum heart rate) than in physiological PCS [34]. This late symptom exacerbation is thought to be due to stress on the vestibular/ocular systems or excessive motion of the cervical spine characteristic of walking/running at higher workloads. Abnormal physical examination findings that point towards a vestibular or ocular pathology, such as smooth pursuits, repetitive saccades, vestibulo-ocular reflex, near point convergence (binocular vision), abnormal accommodation (monocular vision), and benign paroxysmal positional vertigo, are present in almost 70% of patient with mTBI [36, 37]. Clinical predictors of vestibulo-ocular PCS include female sex, pre-injury depression, post-traumatic amnesia, history of motion sickness, dizziness, blurred vision, and difficulty focusing at the time of injury [38, 39]. The neck and suboccipital regions are also frequently involved in head injuries and can cause headaches, persistent dizziness, and balance difficulties [40]. Isolated persistent dysfunction (beyond the normal duration of recovery) may suggest lesions in cranial nerves, their nuclei, or the brain stem, and are associated with prolonged recovery [41]. These overlapping symptoms make the diagnosis of PCS difficult and it is possible that patients with physiological PCS can also have isolated dysfunction in the vestibular, ocular, and cervical systems at the same time.

The last subtype, mood-related PCS, presents with symptoms that are primarily affective and/or cognitive in nature, have minimal physical examination signs, and are capable of exercising to exhaustion without significant symptom exacerbation. The management of this sub-type is challenging, even for an experienced concussion expert, because of the extensive overlap with symptoms of primary mood disorders. The most recent concussion in sport group (CISG) guidelines recommend a multidisciplinary team approach to treatment that may involve a psychiatrist, a psychologist and/or a neuropsychologist [21]. Other disorders, such as chronic post-traumatic headaches and migraines, are treated in a similar fashion and should be referred to their corresponding specialist, i.e., a neurologist.

3. Sex differences

The duration of recovery is suggested to be longer for females with males recovering in an average of 7–10 days where as females recovering in an average of 14 days [21]. Healthy females at baseline are also reported to have higher symptom severity on concussion symptom scales than healthy males [42]. A study [43] suggests that adolescent females were more likely to be diagnosed with PCS due to increased symptom load as well as the duration of symptoms because males returned to being asymptomatic by the fourth week of recovery, missing the PCS diagnostic criteria. Another study suggests the female sex to be a significant predictor of prolonged PCS, which they described as symptoms that lasted for more than 3 months [44]. Interestingly, the same study found this association to be more prominent between the ages of 14 and 56, which is characterized by drastic fluctuations of hormone levels. This calls into question the role of female sex hormones in recovery trajectories and symptom resolution. Some critics have suggested that the above theories overestimate sex effect on PCS, suggesting that the increased relative rates of females entering PCS and experiencing PCS symptoms are more often due to differing societal pressures and perceived stigma experienced by the sexes causing many males to perceive their symptoms as resolved [45, 46].

A topic of more recent research is the morphological and structural differences in females that could predict PCS. It has been well established by the literature that female athletes, given equal exposure and risk, are more likely to sustain a concussion [47]. The reasoning behind a female's increased vulnerability is still under debate, with decreased neck girth and differences in play style all seeming to play a role [48, 49]. A recently [50] identified difference in female brains is decreased axon size and density. This decreased axon size complimented with an increased density of axonal fibers could predispose females to having more severe consequences than males when given the same impact. More research in the cellular differences between males and females could address the differences observed in PCS incidence.

4. Imaging

Currently, the ICD-10 states that no advanced imaging methods can diagnose a concussion [21], but some studies have shown that certain types of PCS have observable differences from each other on advanced imaging. PCS patients with neuropsychiatric complains have significant differences than PCS patients without them. Diffusion tensor imaging (DTI) studies [51] have shown decreased fractional anisotropy (FA) in the superior longitudinal fasciculus, vermis, and white matter around the nucleus accumbens and anterior limb of the internal capsule which correlates to symptoms of depression and anxiety. A larger meta-analysis [52] showed patients who had predominantly cognitive/affective symptoms 1 month post-mTBI had significantly increased FA and reduced mean diffusivity (MD) than those with other symptoms. Increased FA indicates faster unidirectional flow within neurons and decreased MD indicates better axonal integrity [53], which is surprising after the brain is injured. Another way to interpret these findings is that there is more activity within each neuron, which is more consistent with the hypothesized post-mTBI hyper-metabolic state described above. Long-term changes have also been shown to occur after mTBI and PCS. A study [54] that longitudinally assessed regional brain volumes at 1 month post-injury and again at 1 year post-injury. They found significant reductions in the anterior cingulate white matter, left cingulate gyrus isthmus white matter, and right precuneal gray matter. The reduction in left cingulate gyrus isthmus correlated with clinical scores on anxiety and depression, which is a prominent symptom of PCS. Similarly, electrophysiology studies have also provided evidence for this. Electroencephalographic (EEG) studies [55] have shown altered frontal-alpha asymmetry and beta asymmetry in patients who self-reported depression/anxiety and anger post-mTBI respectively. A magneto-encephalography study [56] has reported high accuracy in identifying patients with mTBI, with a much higher reliability for blast injuries. More research is warranted to identify imaging biomarkers that can diagnose mTBI, the different PCS sub-types, as well as their recovery.

5. Autonomic nervous system (ANS) dysfunction and PCS

The Autonomic Nervous System (ANS) control centers are located in the brainstem and can be damaged when rotational forces are applied to the upper cervical spine [57]. This damage has been confirmed in a recent DTI study [58] in patients with PCS, with PCS patient displaying a significantly higher percent high and low voxels upon follow up scan. The ANS dysfunction could be due to damage to these centers are/or due to uncoupling of these centers and cardiovascular system [8, 59]. This may cause reduced heart rate variability, a measure of sympathovagal reactivity. This stunted reactivity has been documented at rest and during exercise in the acute phase after concussions, as well as several months after [60]. Cardiovascular dysfunction in PCS may manifest as symptoms of orthostatic hypotension, postural orthostatic tachycardia syndrome, and altered heart rate and blood pressure responses at rest and during exercise, all which are common in PCS [31]. Studies have also shown abnormal ANS function, as assessed by heart rate variability metrics, when moving from rest to a state of increased metabolic demand in PCS, and this dysfunction can persist even after the patient is clinically recovered [61].

Patients with acute concussions and PCS have also been found to have higher rates of sympathetic nervous system output than controls, as exemplified by higher resting heart rates [62] and higher heart rates during cognitive [63] and physical exercise [64]. A study done on acutely concussed adults showed a blunted parasympathetic response to stimuli, with concussed athletes showing a stunted mean arterial pressure and first-minute high frequency power rise when compared to controls, as well as altogether lack of significant changes in heart rate upon face cooling [65]. This abnormal sympathovagal imbalance may help explain some of the clinical symptoms of PCS. One example is sleep disturbances in PCS because it involves activation of the parasympathetic drive [66]. This increased sympathetic drive may interfere with the onset and maintenance of sleep [67].

6. Cerebral blood flow and PCS

The brain needs a constant perfusion pressure, i.e., the supply of blood and nutrients, irrespective of changes in cerebral blood flow (CBF) or systemic blood pressure. Increases or decreases in CBF are detected by a series of receptors which provide local and systemic responses [68]. Local responses include constriction or dilation of cerebral blood vessels and systemic responses include altering the cardiac contractibility and systemic blood pressure. This protects the brain from changes in sympathetic nerve activity, mean arterial blood pressure, and arterial CO_2 levels [69]. Of relevance to physiological PCS, the ANS controls the CBF response to exercise which is suspected to be the cause of symptom exacerbation on physical exertion [70]. Evidence to support this hypothesis includes lower resting global CBF detected beyond symptom recovery using MR-angiography, with 64% of sport-related concussion patients showing CBF improvements within 30 days [71, 72], and regional alterations in resting CBF in patients with PCS [73–75]. Taken together, there is an abundance of evidence that cerebral autoregulation is impaired in PCS, a likely explanation for many physiological PCS symptoms.

Functional magnetic resonance imaging (fMRI) have also been used to assess patients with concussion and PCS. fMRI can assess task-evoked blood-oxygen-level-dependent (BOLD) responses either during resting state or during cognitive tasks [76]. PCS patients have cognitive intolerance so it logical to assess for differences in activation/inactivation during cognitive tasks. Changes in regional deoxy-hemoglobin concentrations can also been assessed using functional near-infrared spectroscopy (fNIRS) [77]. Abnormal CBF regulation should lead to differences in BOLD responses in the PCS brain so research is currently being done to find objective biomarkers for PCS. Unfortunately, the literature is not decisive [78]. Studies have shown decreased BOLD activity in thalamus and hypothalamus as well as frontal/temporal regions but increased functional connectivity in certain brain circuits including enhanced thalami-cortical functional connectivity based on resting-state BOLD responses in TBI patients in comparison to healthy controls. There could be several reasons for these differences, it could be due to the multiple sub-types of PCS, some causing an increases response whereas other causing a decreased response, or due to the time since injury with acute cases showing more activation due to neuro-metabolic activity and chronic cases showing decreased activity. More research is warranted to understand the pathophysiology of CBF autoregulation disturbances in PCS.

7. Intra-cranial pressure (ICP) and PCS

Intra-cranial pressure (ICP) is the pressure of the cerebrospinal fluid in the subarachnoid space and is between 7 and 15 mmHg in a healthy supine adult and -10 mmHg in the standing position [79]. Since the brain is inside a stiff skull with fixed volume, an increase in ICP could lead to impaired CBF and is an important cause of secondary insult due to ischemia [80, 81]. ICP can be measured using direct and indirect methods. Direct methods, such as intraventricular catheter, are invasive, have high risk of complications and are not justified for mTBI [82]. Indirect methods, like ultrasonographic or ophthalmological, are noninvasive but have a downside of being less sensitive and less reliable [83]. Increased ICP has already been documented in moderate and severe traumatic brain injury (TBI) and their treatment includes monitoring and normalization of the ICP. Due to the mild nature of mTBI, directly measured ICP has not been studied in much detail in this population but there is one systematic review that suggests a prolonged increase in ICP after an mTBI and recommends further research [84]. One particular study [85] of interest used intravenous hypertonic 3% saline on acutely concussed patients. Hypertonic saline is a commonly used pharmacotherapy for treatment of increased ICP and its efficacy has been documented in moderate to severe forms of TBI [81, 86–89]. The study showed a significant decrease in concussion-specific symptoms after an infusion of hypertonic saline but did not measure ICP, hence the

ICP response to hypertonic saline is an assumption. More research needs to be done in PCS to investigate this possible alternate method of treatment.

8. Neuroinflammation

Neuroinflammation is the inflammation of nervous tissue and is present in several pathological conditions such as infection, injury, autoimmunity, toxicity and aging [90]. The central nervous system (CNS) has its own native cells, the microglia and astrocytes, capable of initiating the inflammatory response [91–93]. While neuroinflammation is recognized to promote protective and regenerative effects by activating alternative pathways, persistent neuroinflammation is considered detrimental in several diseases and is an area of interest in several neurodegenerative diseases [94]. Among the several inflammatory mediators released after TBI, some of the most researched include tumor necrosis factor-α (TNFα) [95] and interleukin-1β [96]. TNFα has been shown to be produced early after experimental mTBI, generally returning to baseline levels within 24 hours of injury. Mice with dysfunctional TNFα systems have prolonged recovery (2–3 weeks versus >4 weeks), increased cell damage, and increased blood brain barrier permeability (BBB) with the extent of BBB breach being 0.9mm^3 greater in TNFα receptor lacking mice after TBI [97, 98]. However, the literature on TNFα role in mTBI is controversial. Older studies have shown that inhibition of TNFα after mTBI in animal models can be beneficial by improving neurological outcome, motor function recovery, and decreasing edema size [99, 100]. However, a newer study has shown that TNFα knockout mice performed poorly when compared to wild type mice after concussive brain injury [101]. The authors of that study also concluded that TNFα inhibition influence cognitive deficits independent of mTBI so these therapies are not appropriate for mTBI.

9. Treatment of PCS

Treatment of concussion and PCS has changed significantly over that past decade. The previous standard of care used to be complete physical and cognitive rest with a high degree of social isolation until symptoms resolve [102]. This "rest is best" model of care was supported by evidence that showed that the brain is vulnerable immediately after a concussion with cognitive or physical stress [12] and excessing physical activity [103, 104] would prolong the recovery. Forced aerobic exercise imposed upon rodents within 2 weeks of fluid percussion-simulated concussion was shown to be detrimental to recovery of cognitive function. However, exercise administered three or more weeks after injury in rodents was beneficial to both. A recent randomized controlled trial in humans compared prolonged rest to a short period of rest followed by a step-wise return to activity and found that the strict rest group reported more daily symptoms and a prolonged duration of recovery [105]. Another observational study suggests that moderate levels of physical activity, specifically aerobic exercise, within the first week after injury reduces the incidence of PCS in children and adolescents [15]. This growing body of evidence has changed the management of concussions and PCS and the most recent CISG guidelines [21] recommend a short period of rest (24–48 hours) post-injury, followed by a graded return to sub-threshold activity. There have been more studies [106] that have shown the benefits of early sub-threshold aerobic activity in concussion and PCS since guideline came out. A recent randomized controlled trial [107] of over a hundred acutely concussed adolescents showed a significant reduction in recovery time from a median of 17 days in the placebo group to a median of 13 days in the aerobic exercise group (p = 0.006). This study is a turning point and will affect the approach to concussion treatment worldwide [108].

There are several theories why light to moderate levels of exercise can improve recovery from PCS. The neurocognitive benefits of exercise, such as attenuation of cognitive impairment and reduction of dementia risk in humans, have been known for years [109]. The proposed mechanism of brain health is due to the action of factors that promote neuron growth and repair. Brain derived neurotrophic factor (BDNF) is one of these factors that increase hippocampal volume and improves spatial memory [110]. BDNF levels have been shown to increase after exercise in animals [109] which has provided pre-clinical support for the observation that patients with PPCS recover much faster with sub-threshold aerobic exercise treatment [29]. In humans, studies have shown that exercise increases BDNF level as early as 5–6 weeks after initiation of aerobic training, which has a positive influence on brain neuroplasticity [111, 112]. In regards of CBF regulation, physical deconditioning from prolonged rest has been shown to impair CBF regulation [113], which is already impaired in PCS as discussed above, whereas exercise has been shown to be beneficial in improving CBF regulation [114]. The rapidity of the beneficial effect of exercise on neuroplasticity suggests improved neuronal function rather than reduced cerebrovascular disease risk being the cause for increased brain health and function. An interesting finding is that not all light to moderate exercise causes an increase in BDNF. Rats who were "forced" to exercise after concussion did not increase BDNF levels and showed an increase in stress hormone levels, which was not seen in rats who exercised voluntarily [115, 116]. This emphasizes the benefits of voluntary, sub-symptom threshold exercise during PCS.

Currently, there are no pharmacological therapies that are recommended for PCS [117]. Several pharmacological therapies have been researched but there is not enough empirical evidence to suggest their efficacy. A randomized controlled trial [118] studied the effects of the anti-Parkinson drug, amantadine, in adolescents with PCS and found that it significantly improved symptomology and cognitive function (as assessed by a computerized neurocognitive test). However, more evidence is needed to recommend these therapies. Psychostimulants such as methylphenidate and amphetamines, have been considered as pharmacological therapies for cognitive dysfunction after PCS [117]. This is based on studies that have proven their efficacy in moderate and severe forms of TBI [119–121]. Research is required on patients with mTBI before it can be recommended for PCS.

10. Long-term sequelae

There has been an increase in the awareness of long-term consequences of repetitive concussions and PCS since the discovery of chronic traumatic encephalopathy (CTE) in a retired American football player in 2005 [122]. CTE is a neurodegenerative disorder characterized by significant emotional disturbances, cognitive decline, and deposition of Tau proteins in the brain [123]. The Tau proteinopathy seen in CTE is different from the Tau proteinopathy seen in Alzheimer's disease because it is found widespread in the frontal and temporal lobes [124], as opposed to localization in the limbic system in Alzheimer's. There is no uncertainty that CTE is caused by repetitive head injuries, and has been described as early at 1928 in boxers [125], and the increased awareness of long-term consequences of repetitive head injuries, concussive or sub-concussive, have made it a popular topic in the media and research. The National Institutes of Health held a consensus meeting in 2016 with the aim of defining the neuropathological criteria for CTE diagnosis [126].

They blindly evaluated 25 cases of various tau proteinopathies, including CTE and a number of dementing brain diseases, and the results demonstrated reasonably good agreement and improved specificity to the diagnosis of CTE.

There is some controversy in the incidence rate of CTE and if the presence of tau protein represents trauma-induced CTE versus normal deposits as a result of age and other life factors [127]. Some researchers suggest a very high incidence of CTE in anyone who participated in a contact sport, with rates as high as 75–99% [124, 128]. All of these studies have been done by post-mortem analysis of brain tissue, which is currently the only way to definitely diagnose CTE [129]. However, several studies have been performed since 2017 which have brought uncertainty to the clinical manifestations and incidence of CTE, i.e., the patterns of behavior and cognitive deficits experienced by the living individual affected by CTE. Retired contact-sport athletes have be shown to have no differences in cognition [130, 131], mild cognitive impairment [132], executive function [133], or structural or functional brain differences [134]. This suggests that although Tau proteins may deposit in the brain after head-injuries, they do not causes significant decrease in function unless it is very severe.

11. Conclusion

PCS is a complex disorder and its pathophysiology is not clearly understood. There are no symptoms, or group of symptoms, that can accurately diagnose PCS. Females may be at a higher risk of developing PCS than male. Although there are no advanced imaging biomarkers for PCS, some studies present differences in those patients who predominantly complain of mood-related or cognitive symptoms when compared with other sub-types of PCS. Longitudinal changes in the brain have been identified in PCS up to 1 year since concussive head injury. ANS dysfunction is observed in PCS, which could be due to damage to the ANS control centers located in the hindbrain or uncoupling of the connections between the central ANS and cardiovascular system. Abnormal cardiovascular metrics suggest ANS dysfunction and impaired CBF regulation, which may explain the characteristic finding of symptom-limited exercise intolerance in physiological PCS. Functional imaging, like fMRI, has shown differences between healthy people and patients with PCS, but these differences are not consistent in the literature. Long term consequences of PCS or repetitive concussions include CTE, but the clinical manifestations of CTE need to be studied in greater detail. Therapies for PCS include sub-threshold aerobic exercise, which may increase neuroplasticity and decrease neuroinflammation through release of BDNF. More research needs to be done to identify objective biomarkers of concussion, PCS, and recovery, as well as therapies for PCS.

Acknowledgements

Research reported in this publication was supported by the National Institute of Neurological Disorders and Stroke of the National Institutes of Health under award number 1R01NS094444. The content is solely the responsibility of the authors and does not necessarily represent the official views of the National Institutes of Health.

Conflict of interest

The author does not declare any conflicts of interest.

Author details

Mohammad Nadir Haider[1]* and Itai Bezherano[2]

1 Department of Orthopedics and Sports Medicine, Concussion Management Clinic and Research Center, State University of New York at Buffalo, Buffalo, NY, USA

2 Department of Exercise and Nutrition Sciences, School of Public Health and Health Professions, State University of New York at Buffalo, Buffalo, NY, USA

*Address all correspondence to: haider@buffalo.edu

References

[1] Signoretti S, Lazzarino G, Tavazzi B, Vagnozzi R. The pathophysiology of concussion. PM & R: The Journal of Injury, Function, and Rehabilitation. 2011;**3**(10):S359-S368

[2] Choe MC. The pathophysiology of concussion. Current Pain and Headache Reports. 2016;**20**(6):42

[3] Anderson T, Heitger M, Macleod A. Concussion and mild head injury. Practical Neurology. 2006;**6**(6):342-357

[4] Cassidy JD, Carroll L, Peloso P, et al. Incidence, risk factors and prevention of mild traumatic brain injury: Results of the WHO collaborating centre task force on mild traumatic brain injury. Journal Rehabilitation Medicine. 2004;**36**(0):28-60

[5] Corrigan JD, Selassie AW, Orman JAL. The epidemiology of traumatic brain injury. The Journal of head trauma rehabilitation. 2010;**25**(2):72-80

[6] Conder RL, Conder AA. Sports-related concussions. North Carolina Medical Journal. 2015;**76**(2):89-95

[7] Tweedie D, Rachmany L, Rubovitch V, et al. Blast traumatic brain injury-induced cognitive deficits are attenuated by preinjury or postinjury treatment with the glucagon-like peptide-1 receptor agonist, exendin-4. Alzheimer's & Dementia. 2016;**12**(1):34-48

[8] Len T, Neary J. Cerebrovascular pathophysiology following mild traumatic brain injury. Clinical Physiology and Functional Imaging. 2011;**31**(2):85-93

[9] Mullally WJ. Concussion. The American Journal of Medicine. 2017;**130**(8):885-892

[10] Dashnaw ML, Petraglia AL, Bailes JE. An overview of the basic science of concussion and subconcussion: Where we are and where we are going. Neurosurgical Focus. 2012;**33**(6):E5:1-E5:9

[11] Petraglia AL, Plog BA, Dayawansa S, et al. The pathophysiology underlying repetitive mild traumatic brain injury in a novel mouse model of chronic traumatic encephalopathy. Surgical Neurology International. 2014;**5**:184

[12] Giza CC, Hovda DA. The new neurometabolic cascade of concussion. Neurosurgery. 2014;**75**(suppl_4):S24-S33

[13] Hill CS, Coleman MP, Menon DK. Traumatic axonal injury: Mechanisms and translational opportunities. Trends in Neurosciences. 2016;**39**(5):311-324

[14] Williams RM, Puetz TW, Giza CC, Broglio SP. Concussion recovery time among high school and collegiate athletes: A systematic review and meta-analysis. Sports Medicine. 2015;**45**(6):893-903

[15] Grool AM, Aglipay M, Momoli F, et al. Association between early participation in physical activity following acute concussion and persistent postconcussive symptoms in children and adolescents. Journal of the American Medical Association. 2016;**316**(23):2504-2514

[16] Jotwani V, Harmon KG. Postconcussion syndrome in athletes. Current Sports Medicine Reports. 2010;**9**(1):21-26

[17] Prigatano GP, Gale SD. The current status of postconcussion syndrome. Current Opinion in Psychiatry. 2011;**24**(3):243-250

[18] Tator CH, Davis HS, Dufort PA, et al. Postconcussion syndrome: Demographics and predictors in 221

patients. Journal of Neurosurgery. 2016;**125**(5):1206-1216

[19] Iverson GL, Lange RT. Post-concussion syndrome. In: The Little Black Book of Neuropsychology. New York, USA: Springer; 2011. pp. 745-763

[20] Arciniegas DB, Anderson CA, Topkoff J, McAllister TW. Mild traumatic brain injury: A neuropsychiatric approach to diagnosis, evaluation, and treatment. Neuropsychiatric Disease and Treatment. 2005;**1**(4):311-327

[21] McCrory P, Meeuwisse W, Dvorak J, et al. Consensus statement on concussion in sport—The 5th international conference on concussion in sport held in Berlin, October 2016. British Journal of Sports Medicine. 2017;**51**(11):838-847

[22] Haider MN, Leddy JJ, Pavlesen S, et al. A systematic review of criteria used to define recovery from sport-related concussion in youth athletes. British Journal of Sports Medicine. 2017. DOI: 10.1136/bjsports-2016-096551

[23] Organization WH. The ICD-10 Classification of Mental and Behavioural Disorders: Clinical Descriptions and Diagnostic Guidelines. Geneva: World Health Organization; 1992

[24] Echemendia RJ, Meeuwisse W, McCrory P, et al. The sport concussion assessment tool 5th edition (SCAT5). British Journal of Sports Medicine. 2017;**51**(11):848-850. DOI: 10.1136/bjsports-2017-097506

[25] McCrory P, Meeuwisse W, Johnston K, et al. SCAT2. British Journal of Sports Medicine. 2009;**43**(Suppl_1):i85-i88

[26] Dean PJ, O'Neill D, Sterr A. Post-concussion syndrome: Prevalence after mild traumatic brain injury in comparison with a sample without head injury. Brain Injury. 2012;**26**(1):14-26

[27] Kroshus E, Garnett B, Hawrilenko M, Baugh CM, Calzo JP. Concussion under-reporting and pressure from coaches, teammates, fans, and parents. Social Science and Medicine. 2015;**134**:66-75

[28] Althubaiti A. Information bias in health research: Definition, pitfalls, and adjustment methods. Journal of Multidisciplinary Healthcare. 2016;**9**:211-217

[29] Leddy JJ, Kozlowski K, Donnelly JP, Pendergast DR, Epstein LH, Willer B. A preliminary study of subsymptom threshold exercise training for refractory post-concussion syndrome. Clinical Journal of Sport Medicine. 2010;**20**(1):21-27

[30] Gioia G, Schneider J, Vaughan C, Isquith P. Which symptom assessments and approaches are uniquely appropriate for paediatric concussion? British Journal of Sports Medicine. 2009;**43**(Suppl 1):i13-i22

[31] Matuszak JM, McVige J, McPherson J, Willer B, Leddy J. A Practical concussion physical examination toolbox evidence-based physical examination for concussion. Sports Health: A Multidisciplinary Approach. 2016;**8**(3):260-269

[32] Haider MN, Leddy JJ, Du W, Viera K, Willer B. Practical Management: Brief physical examination for sport-related concussion in the outpatient setting. Clinical Journal of Sport Medicine. 2018. [Epub ahead of print]

[33] Fife TD, Giza C. Posttraumatic vertigo and dizziness. In: Paper presented at: Seminars in Neurology. 2013

[34] Kozlowski KF, Graham J, Leddy JJ, Devinney-Boymel L, Willer BS. Exercise intolerance in individuals with postconcussion syndrome. Journal of Athletic Training. 2013;**48**(5):627-635

[35] Silver JM, McAllister TW, Archiniegas DB. Textbook of Traumatic Brain Injury. 3nd ed. Washington, DC: American Psychiatric Pub; 2019

[36] Master CL, Scheiman M, Gallaway M, et al. Vision diagnoses are common after concussion in adolescents. Clinical Pediatrics (Phila). 2016;**55**(3):260-267

[37] Ventura RE, Balcer LJ, Galetta SL. The neuro-ophthalmology of head trauma. The Lancet Neurology. 2014;**13**(10):1006-1016

[38] Ellis MJ, Cordingley DM, Vis S, Reimer KM, Leiter J, Russell K. Clinical predictors of vestibulo-ocular dysfunction in pediatric sports-related concussion. Journal of Neurosurgery Pediatrics. 2017;**19**(1):38-45

[39] Kontos AP, Sufrinko A, Elbin RJ, Puskar A, Collins MW. Reliability and associated risk factors for performance on the vestibular/ocular motor screening (VOMS) tool in healthy collegiate athletes. The American Journal of Sports Medicine. 2016;**44**(6):1400-1406

[40] Marshall CM, Vernon H, Leddy JJ, Baldwin BA. The role of the cervical spine in post-concussion syndrome. The Physician and sportsmedicine. 2015;**43**(3):274-284

[41] Anzalone AJ, Blueitt D, Case T, et al. A positive vestibular/ocular motor screening (VOMS) is associated with increased recovery time after sports-related concussion in youth and adolescent athletes. The American Journal of Sports Medicine. 2017;**45**(2):474-479

[42] Brown DA, Elsass JA, Miller AJ, Reed LE, Reneker JC. Differences in symptom reporting between males and females at baseline and after a sports-related concussion: A systematic review and meta-analysis. Sports Medicine. 2015;**45**(7):1027-1040

[43] Henry LC, Elbin RJ, Collins MW, Marchetti G, Kontos AP. Examining recovery trajectories after sport-related concussion with a multimodal clinical assessment approach. Neurosurgery. 2016;**78**(2):232-241

[44] Bazarian JJ, Blyth B, Mookerjee S, He H, McDermott MP. Sex differences in outcome after mild traumatic brain injury. Journal of Neurotrauma. 2010;**27**(3):527-539

[45] Laker SR. Epidemiology of concussion and mild traumatic brain injury. PM & R: The Journal of Injury, Function, and Rehabilitation. 2011;**3**(10 Suppl 2):S354-S358

[46] Wallace J, Covassin T, Beidler E. Sex differences in high school athletes' knowledge of sport-related concussion symptoms and reporting behaviors. Journal of Athletic Training. 2017;**52**(7):682-688

[47] Roos KG, Wasserman EB, Dalton SL, et al. Epidemiology of 3825 injuries sustained in six seasons of national collegiate athletic association men's and women's soccer (2009/2010-2014/2015). British Journal of Sports Medicine. 2017;**51**(13):1029-1034

[48] Bretzin AC, Mansell JL, Tierney RT, McDevitt JK. Sex differences in anthropometrics and heading kinematics among division I soccer athletes. Sports Health. 2017;**9**(2):168-173

[49] Chandran A, Barron MJ, Westerman BJ, DiPietro L. Multifactorial examination of sex-differences in head injuries and concussions among collegiate soccer players: NCAA ISS, 2004-2009. Injury Epidemiology. 2017;**4**(1):28

[50] Dollé J-P, Jaye A, Anderson SA, Ahmadzadeh H, Shenoy VB, Smith DH. Newfound sex differences in axonal structure underlie differential

outcomes from in vitro traumatic axonal injury. Experimental Neurology. 2018;**300**:121-134

[51] Alhilali LM, Delic JA, Gumus S, Fakhran S. Evaluation of white matter injury patterns underlying neuropsychiatric symptoms after mild traumatic brain injury. Radiology. 2015;**277**(3):793-800

[52] Aoki Y, Inokuchi R, Gunshin M, Yahagi N, Suwa H. Diffusion tensor imaging studies of mild traumatic brain injury: A meta-analysis. Journal of Neurology, Neurosurgery, and Psychiatry. 2012;**83**(9):870-876

[53] Cubon VA, Putukian M, Boyer C. Dettwiler a. A diffusion tensor imaging study on the white matter skeleton in individuals with sports-related concussion. Journal of Neurotrauma. 2011;**28**(2):189-201

[54] Zhou Y, Kierans A, Kenul D, et al. Mild traumatic brain injury: Longitudinal regional brain volume changes. Radiology. 2013;**267**(3):880-890

[55] Moore RD, Sauve W, Ellemberg D. Neurophysiological correlates of persistent psycho-affective alterations in athletes with a history of concussion. Brain Imaging and Behavior. 2015;**10**(4):1108-1116

[56] Huang M-X, Nichols S, Robb A, et al. An automatic MEG low-frequency source imaging approach for detecting injuries in mild and moderate TBI patients with blast and non-blast causes. NeuroImage. 2012;**61**(4):1067-1082

[57] Ivancevic VG. New mechanics of traumatic brain injury. Cognitive Neurodynamics. 2009;**3**(3):281

[58] Polak P, Leddy JJ, Dwyer MG, Willer B, Zivadinov R. Diffusion tensor imaging alterations in patients with postconcussion syndrome undergoing exercise treatment: A pilot longitudinal study. The Journal of head trauma rehabilitation. 2015;**30**(2):E32-E42

[59] La Fountaine MF, Heffernan KS, Gossett JD, Bauman WA, De Meersman RE. Transient suppression of heart rate complexity in concussed athletes. Autonomic Neuroscience. 2009;**148**(1-2):101-103

[60] Abaji JP, Curnier D, Moore RD, Ellemberg D. Persisting effects of concussion on heart rate variability during physical exertion. Journal of Neurotrauma. 2016;**33**(9):811-817

[61] Kamins J, Bigler E, Covassin T, et al. What is the physiological time to recovery after concussion? Systematic Review. British Journal of Sports Medicine. 2017;**51**(12):935-940. DOI: 10.1136/bjsports-2016-097464

[62] Ellis MJ, Leddy JJ, Willer B. Physiological, vestibulo-ocular and cervicogenic post-concussion disorders: An evidence-based classification system with directions for treatment. Brain Injury. 2015;**29**(2):238-248

[63] Hanna-Pladdy B, Berry ZM, Bennett T, Phillips HL, Gouvier WD. Stress as a diagnostic challenge for postconcussive symptoms: Sequelae of mild traumatic brain injury or physiological stress response. The Clinical Neuropsychologist. 2001;**15**(3):289-304

[64] Gall B, Parkhouse W, Goodman D. Exercise following a sport induced concussion. British Journal of Sports Medicine. 2004;**38**(6):773-777

[65] Johnson BD, O'Leary MC, McBryde M, Sackett JR, Schlader ZJ, Leddy JJ. Face cooling exposes cardiac parasympathetic and sympathetic dysfunction in recently concussed college athletes. Physiological Reports. 2018;**6**(9):e13694

[66] Minen MT, Boubour A, Walia H, Barr W. Post-concussive syndrome:

A focus on post-traumatic headache and related cognitive, psychiatric, and sleep issues. Current Neurology and Neuroscience Reports. 2016;**16**(11):100

[67] El-Sheikh M, Erath SA, Bagley EJ. Parasympathetic nervous system activity and children's sleep. Journal of Sleep Research. 2013;**22**(3):282-288

[68] Zamir M, Moir ME, Klassen SA, Balestrini CS, Shoemaker JK. Cerebrovascular compliance within the rigid confines of the skull. Frontiers in Physiology. 2018;**9**

[69] Clausen M, Pendergast DR, Wilier B, Leddy J. Cerebral blood flow during treadmill exercise is a marker of physiological postconcussion syndrome in female athletes. The Journal of Head Trauma Rehabilitation. 2016;**31**(3):215-224

[70] Epps C, Allen M. Neurovascular coupling: A unifying theory for post-concussion syndrome treatment and functional neuroimaging. Journal of Neurology and Neurophysiology. 2017;**8**(454):2

[71] Maugans TA, Farley C, Altaye M, Leach J, Cecil KM. Pediatric sports-related concussion produces cerebral blood flow alterations. Pediatrics. 2012;**129**(1):28-37

[72] Meier TB, Bellgowan PS, Singh R, Kuplicki R, Polanski DW, Mayer AR. Recovery of cerebral blood flow following sports-related concussion. Journal of the American Medical Association Neurology. 2015;**72**(5):530-538

[73] Ellis MJ, Ryner L, Sobczyk O, et al. Neuroimaging assessment of cerebrovascular reactivity in concussion: current concepts, methodological considerations, and review of the literature. Frontiers of Neurology. 2016;**7**:61

[74] Mutch WA, Ellis MJ, Graham MR, et al. Brain MRI CO_2 stress testing: A pilot study in patients with concussion. PLoS One. 2014;**9**(7):e102181

[75] Mutch WA, Ellis MJ, Ryner LN, et al. Longitudinal brain magnetic resonance imaging CO_2 stress testing in individual adolescent sports-related concussion patients: A pilot study. Frontiers in Neurology. 2016;**7**:107

[76] Glover GH. Overview of functional magnetic resonance imaging. Neurosurgery Clinics. 2011;**22**(2):133-139

[77] Kontos A, Huppert T, Beluk N, et al. Brain activation during neurocognitive testing using functional near-infrared spectroscopy in patients following concussion compared to healthy controls. Brain Imaging and Behavior. 2014;**8**(4):621-634

[78] McDonald BC, Saykin AJ, McAllister TW. Functional MRI of mild traumatic brain injury (mTBI): Progress and perspectives from the first decade of studies. Brain Imaging and Behavior. 2012;**6**(2):193-207

[79] Czosnyka M, Pickard JD. Monitoring and interpretation of intracranial pressure. Journal of Neurology, Neurosurgery and Psychiatry. 2004;**75**(6):813-821

[80] Steiner L, Andrews P. Monitoring the injured brain: ICP and CBF. British Journal of Anaesthesia. 2006;**97**(1):26-38

[81] Czosnyka M, Pickard J, Steiner L. Principles of intracranial pressure monitoring and treatment. Handbook of Clinical Neurology. 2017;**140**:67

[82] Muralidharan R. External ventricular drains: Management and complications. Surgical Neurology International. 2015;**6**(Suppl 6):S271

[83] Kristiansson H, Nissborg E, Bartek J Jr, Andresen M, Reinstrup P, Romner B. Measuring elevated intracranial pressure through noninvasive methods: A review of the literature. Journal of Neurosurgical Anesthesiology. 2013;**25**(4):372-385

[84] Haider MN, Leddy JJ, Hinds AL, et al. Intracranial pressure changes after mild traumatic brain injury: A systematic review. Brain Injury. 2018;**32**(7):809-815

[85] Lumba-Brown A, Harley J, Lucio S, Vaida F, Hilfiker M. Hypertonic saline as a therapy for pediatric concussive pain: A randomized controlled trial of symptom treatment in the emergency department. Pediatric Emergency Care. 2014;**30**(3):139-145

[86] Maguigan KL, Dennis BM, Hamblin SE, Guillamondegui OD. Method of hypertonic saline administration: Effects on osmolality in traumatic brain injury patients. Journal of Clinical Neuroscience. 2017;**39**:147-150

[87] Sokhal N, Rath GP, Chaturvedi A, Singh M, Dash HH. Comparison of 20% mannitol and 3% hypertonic saline on intracranial pressure and systemic hemodynamics. Journal of Clinical Neuroscience. 2017

[88] Johnson AL, Criddle LM. Pass the salt indications for and implications of using hypertonic saline. Critical Care Nurse. 2004;**24**(5):36-48

[89] Rockswold GL, Solid CA, Paredes-Andrade E, Rockswold SB, Jancik JT, Quickel RR. Hypertonic saline and its effect on intracranial pressure, cerebral perfusion pressure, and brain tissue oxygen. Neurosurgery. 2009;**65**(6):1035-1042

[90] Ransohoff RM, Schafer D, Vincent A, Blachère NE, Bar-Or A. Neuroinflammation: Ways in which the immune system affects the brain. Neurotherapeutics. 2015;**12**(4):896-909

[91] Wang X, Feuerstein GZ. Role of immune and inflammatory mediators in CNS injury. Drug News & Perspectives. 2000;**13**(3):133-140

[92] Szmydynger-Chodobska J, Strazielle N, Gandy JR, et al. Posttraumatic invasion of monocytes across the blood—Cerebrospinal fluid barrier. Journal of Cerebral Blood Flow and Metabolism. 2012;**32**(1):93-104

[93] Singh S, Swarnkar S, Goswami P, Nath C. Astrocytes and microglia: Responses to neuropathological conditions. International Journal of Neuroscience. 2011;**121**(11):589-597

[94] Frankola K, Greig N, Luo W, Tweedie D. Targeting TNF-alpha to elucidate and ameliorate neuroinflammation in neurodegenerative diseases. CNS & Neurological Disorders-Drug Targets. 2011;**10**(3):391-403

[95] Patterson ZR, Holahan MR. Understanding the neuroinflammatory response following concussion to develop treatment strategies. Frontiers in Cellular Neuroscience. 2012;**6**

[96] Taib T, Leconte C, Van Steenwinckel J, et al. Neuroinflammation, myelin and behavior: Temporal patterns following mild traumatic brain injury in mice. PLoS One. 2017;**12**(9):e0184811

[97] Scherbel U, Raghupathi R, Nakamura M, et al. Differential acute and chronic responses of tumor necrosis factor-deficient mice to experimental brain injury. Proceedings of the National Academy of Sciences. 1999;**96**(15):8721-8726

[98] Sullivan PG, Bruce-Keller AJ, Rabchevsky AG, et al. Exacerbation of damage and altered NF-κB activation in mice lacking tumor necrosis factor receptors after traumatic brain injury. Journal of Neuroscience. 1999;**19**(15):6248-6256

[99] Shohami E, Bass R, Wallach D, Yamin A, Gallily R. Inhibition of tumor necrosis factor alpha (TNFα) activity in rat brain is associated with cerebroprotection after closed head injury. Journal of Cerebral Blood Flow and Metabolism. 1996;**16**(3):378-384

[100] Shohami E, Gallily R, Mechoulam R, Bass R, Ben-Hur T. Cytokine production in the brain following closed head injury: Dexanabinol (HU-211) is a novel TNF-α inhibitor and an effective neuroprotectant. Journal of Neuroimmunology. 1997;**72**(2):169-177

[101] Khuman J, Meehan IIIWP, Zhu X, et al. Tumor necrosis factor alpha and Fas receptor contribute to cognitive deficits independent of cell death after concussive traumatic brain injury in mice. Journal of Cerebral Blood Flow and Metabolism. 2011;**31**(2):778-789

[102] McCrory P, Meeuwisse WH, Aubry M, et al. Consensus statement on concussion in sport: The 4th international conference on concussion in sport held in Zurich, November 2012. British Journal of Sports Medicine. 2013;**47**(5):250-258

[103] Griesbach GS, Hovda DA, Molteni R, Wu A, Gomez-Pinilla F. Voluntary exercise following traumatic brain injury: Brain-derived neurotrophic factor upregulation and recovery of function. Neuroscience. 2004;**125**(1):129-139

[104] Majerske CW, Mihalik JP, Ren D, et al. Concussion in sports: Postconcussive activity levels, symptoms, and neurocognitive performance. Journal of Athletic Training. 2008;**43**(3):265-274

[105] Thomas DG, Apps JN, Hoffmann RG, McCrea M, Hammeke T. Benefits of strict rest after acute concussion: A randomized controlled trial. Pediatrics. 2015;**135**(2):213-223

[106] Leddy JJ, Haider MN, Hinds AL, Darling S, Willer BSA. Preliminary study of the effect of early aerobic exercise treatment for sport-related concussion in males. Clinical Journal of Sport Medicine. 2018; Published Online

[107] Leddy JJ, Haider MN, Ellis MJ, et al. Early subthreshold aerobic exercise for sport-related concussion: A randomized clinical trial. JAMA Pediatrics. 2019 [Epub ahead of print]

[108] Chrisman SP. Exercise and recovery time for youth with concussions. Journal of the American Medical Association Pediatrics. 2019

[109] Ahlskog JE, Geda YE, Graff-Radford NR, Petersen RC. Physical exercise as a preventive or disease-modifying treatment of dementia and brain aging. Mayo Clinic Proceedings. 2011;**86**(9):876-884

[110] Erickson KI, Voss MW, Prakash RS, et al. Exercise training increases size of hippocampus and improves memory. Proceedings of the National Academy of Sciences of the United States of America. 2011;**108**(7):3017-3022

[111] Stroth S, Hille K, Spitzer M, Reinhardt R. Aerobic endurance exercise benefits memory and affect in young adults. Neuropsychological Rehabilitation. 2009;**19**(2):223-243

[112] Griffin EW, Mullally S, Foley C, Warmington SA, O'Mara SM, Kelly AM. Aerobic exercise improves hippocampal function and increases BDNF in the serum of young adult males. Physiology & Behavior. 2011;**104**(5):934-941

[113] Coupe M, Fortrat J, Larina I, Gauquelin-Koch G, Gharib C, Custaud M. Cardiovascular deconditioning: From autonomic nervous system to microvascular dysfunctions. Respiratory Physiology & Neurobiology. 2009;**169**:S10-S12

[114] Tan CO, Meehan WP 3rd, Iverson GL, Taylor JA. Cerebrovascular regulation, exercise, and mild traumatic brain injury. Neurology. 2014;**83**(18):1665-1672

[115] Griesbach GS, Tio DL, Nair S, Hovda DA. Recovery of stress response coincides with responsiveness to voluntary exercise after traumatic brain injury. Journal of Neurotrauma. 2014;**31**(7):674-682

[116] Griesbach GS, Tio DL, Vincelli J, McArthur DL, Taylor AN. Differential effects of voluntary and forced exercise on stress responses after traumatic brain injury. Journal of Neurotrauma. 2012;**29**(7):1426-1433

[117] Meehan WP. Medical therapies for concussion. Clinics in Sports Medicine. 2011;**30**(1):115-124

[118] Reddy CC, Collins M, Lovell M, Kontos AP. Efficacy of amantadine treatment on symptoms and neurocognitive performance among adolescents following sports-related concussion. The Journal of head trauma rehabilitation. 2013;**28**(4):260-265

[119] Williams SE, Ris MD, Ayyangar R, Schefft B, Berch D. Recovery in pediatric brain injury: Is psychostimulant medication beneficial? The Journal of Head Trauma Rehabilitation. 1998;**13**(3):73-81

[120] Plenger PM, Dixon CE, Castillo RM, Frankowski RF, Yablon SA, Levin HS. Subacute methylphenidate treatment for moderate to moderately severe traumatic brain injury: A preliminary double-blind placebo-controlled study. Archives of Physical Medicine and Rehabilitation. 1996;**77**(6):536-540

[121] Pangilinan PH, Giacoletti-Argento A, Shellhaas R, Hurvitz EA, Hornyak JE. Neuropharmacology in pediatric brain injury: A review. PM & R: The Journal of Injury, Function, and Rehabilitation. 2010;**2**(12):1127-1140

[122] Omalu BI, DeKosky ST, Minster RL, Kamboh MI, Hamilton RL, Wecht CH. Chronic traumatic encephalopathy in a national football league player. Neurosurgery. 2005;**57**(1):128-134

[123] Armstrong RA, McKee AC, Alvarez VE, Cairns NJ. Clustering of tau-immunoreactive pathology in chronic traumatic encephalopathy. Journal of Neural Transmission. 2017;**124**(2):185-192

[124] McKee AC, Stein TD, Nowinski CJ, et al. The spectrum of disease in chronic traumatic encephalopathy. Brain: A Journal of Neurology. 2013;**136**(1):43-64

[125] Martland HS. Punch drunk. Journal of the American Medical Association. 1928;**91**(15):1103-1107

[126] McKee AC, Cairns NJ, Dickson DW, et al. The first NINDS/NIBIB consensus meeting to define neuropathological criteria for the diagnosis of chronic traumatic encephalopathy. Acta Neuropathologica. 2016;**131**(1):75-86

[127] Davis GA, Castellani RJ, McCrory P. Neurodegeneration and sport. Neurosurgery. 2015;**76**(6):643-655; discussion 655-646

[128] Mez J, Daneshvar DH, Kiernan PT, et al. Clinicopathological evaluation of chronic traumatic encephalopathy in players of American football. Journal of the American Medical Association. 2017;**318**(4):360-370

[129] Riley DO, Robbins CA, Cantu RC, Stern RA. Chronic traumatic encephalopathy: Contributions from the Boston University Center for the study of traumatic encephalopathy. Brain Injury. 2015;**29**(2):154-163

[130] Esopenko C, Chow TW, Tartaglia MC, et al. Cognitive and psychosocial

function in retired professional hockey players. Journal of Neurology, Neurosurgery, and Psychiatry. 2017;**88**:512-519. DOI: 10.1136/jnnp-2016-315260

[131] McMillan TM, McSkimming P, Wainman-Lefley J, et al. Long-term health outcomes after exposure to repeated concussion in elite level: Rugby union players. Journal of Neurology, Neurosurgery, and Psychiatry. 2017;**88**(6):505-511

[132] Baker JG, Leddy JJ, Hinds AL, et al. An exploratory study of mild cognitive impairment of retired professional contact sport athletes. The Journal of Head Trauma Rehabilitation. 2018;**33**(5):E16-E23

[133] Willer BS, Tiso MR, Haider MN, et al. Evaluation of executive function and mental health in retired contact sport athletes. The Journal of Head Trauma Rehabilitation. 2018;**33**(5):E9-E15

[134] Zivadinov R, Polak P, Schweser F, et al. Multimodal imaging of retired professional contact sport athletes does not provide evidence of structural and functional brain damage. The Journal of Head Trauma Rehabilitation. 2018;**33**(5):E24-E32

Chapter 2

Neuroprotection, Photoperiod, and Sleep

Marina Martinez-Vargas, Mercedes Graciela Porras-Villalobos, Francisco Estrada-Rojo, Ricardo Jesus Martinez-Tapia, Adan Perez-Arredondo, Antonio Barajas-Martinez and Luz Navarro

Abstract

After an acquired brain injury, responses that induce cell death are activated; however, neuroprotective mechanisms are also activated. The relation between these responses determines the destination of the damaged tissue. This relation presents variations throughout the day; numerous studies have shown that the onset of a stroke occurs preferably in the morning. In the rat, ischemia causes more damage when it is induced during the night. The damage caused by a traumatic brain injury (TBI), in the rat, varies depending on the time of day it is induced. Minor behavioral damage has been reported when the TBI occurs during the night, a period that coincides with the wakefulness of the rat. It also has been observed that sleep deprivation accelerates the recovery. Our group has documented that this is due, in part, to a difference in the degree of activation of cannabinergic, GABAergyc, and glutamatergic systems.

Keywords: circadian rhythm, sleep deprivation, traumatic brain injury, stroke, cannabinergic system, glutamatergic system, GABAergyc system

1. Introduction

Recent research on acquired brain injury, the pathophysiological processes involved, as well as the mechanisms of morphological and functional recovery, have led, among other essential aspects, to the concept of neuroprotection [1]. This term refers to the use of any therapeutic modality that prevents or delays cell death resulting from a neuronal injury. In this sense, neuroprotection could be considered as a cytoprotection technique similar to cardioprotection or vasoprotection [2, 3].

Also, the term neuroprotection has been used to refer to self-protective responses that the body displays when it undergoes an acquired brain injury and tries to maintain the integrity and functionality of the brain [4]. The management of the term neuroprotection, in this sense, is more recent and emphasizes the balance of the body's responses to an event of ischemia and/or traumatic brain injury (TBI).

In a TBI, two types of lesions can be identified. The primary lesion, which corresponds to mechanical damage to the parenchyma or the vasculature, occurs at the moment of impact and is not reversible or curable and the secondary lesion, which corresponds to late effects, which occur hours to days post-trauma, involves a series of functional, structural, cellular, and molecular changes that cause neuronal damage. Among the events that occur, ischemia has been described. When the flow of blood to the brain tissue ceases, the entry of oxygen and nutrients and the exit of potentially toxic metabolites are severely damaged, resulting in biochemical changes in the affected brain area. There is a depletion of glucose and glycogen and failure of Na/K ATPase and other pumps, which result in a decrease in excitation threshold, presence of action potentials, release of excitatory neurotransmitters such as glutamate, massive entry of calcium, and activation of proteases, lipases, and nucleases, among other enzymes [5]. However, as mentioned earlier, neuroprotective responses are also induced; for example, the GABAergic and cannabinergic systems are activated [6, 7]. The balance between both responses will determine the outcome of the damaged tissue [4].

Indeed, the release of glutamate and the activation of its ionotropic receptors are the main events that result in cell death as a consequence of a TBI or cerebral ischemic attack with acute hypoxia [8–10]. The increase in GABAergic synaptic transmission may have neuroprotective effects against cerebral ischemia, and its inhibition increases the alterations induced by this event, while the inhibition of excitatory signals or excitatory neurotransmitters results in the cytoprotection of ischemic brain tissue [6, 11]. GABA mimetic drugs have a protective effect. Thus, administration of GABAA agonists such as benzodiazepines or muscimol attenuates the damage produced by a TBI [12, 13], while bicuculline, a GABAA antagonist, increases it [12].

In vitro and *in vivo* data suggest that the cannabinergic system is a component of mammalian neuroprotective mechanisms that an organism displays after suffering an insult such as a TBI [7, 14–17]. Endocannabinoid anandamide and 2-arachidonoylglycerol (2-Ag) increase after an acquired brain injury [14, 15] and serve as signaling mediators in integrating inhibitory and excitatory synaptic transmission, as they could regulate glutamate and GABA release [17]. Besides, recently it has been reported that 2-Ag keeps brain homeostasis by exerting anti-inflammatory effects in response to harmful insults [17].

2. Neuroprotection and photoperiod

The cerebral ischemic attack, similar to the heart attack, has a marked diurnal rhythm. Numerous studies have shown that the time of onset of cerebral vascular accidents, as well as transient ischemic attacks, occurs preferably between 6:00 and 12:00 h in the morning that is, after the subject gets up and begins to present activity [18–20]. Numerous variables have been mentioned as responsible for this circadian pattern, among which are postural changes, circadian variations of platelet aggregation, thrombolysis, blood pressure, cardiac rhythm, and circulating concentrations of catecholamines, whose maximum levels occur just in this period. In the rat, ischemia causes more significant damage if it is induced in the hours of darkness compared to the hours of light [21].

Our group has analyzed the severity of a TBI concerning the photoperiod. Using the rat as a model, we have found that the recovery from a TBI induced by the technique of "closed head injury" presents diurnal variations, recovery being better if the trauma occurs in the hours of darkness concerning daylight hours [22–24]. In other words, there seems to be a greater neuroprotection response in the hours of darkness. The fact that the functionality of the brain is not the same in the hours of light as in the hours of darkness is not surprising; many pieces of evidence indicate the importance of rhythms in general, and in particular of the circadian rhythms in physiology. The presence of circadian rhythms has been explained as an adaptive response of the different organisms to the environmental variables. All species from cyanobacteria to humans have these rhythms that serve to anticipate the daily variations of different variables such as temperature, light, or food intake. It is accepted that virtually any physiological parameter that has been measured for a period of 24 h in humans has fluctuations [25, 26]. Several aspects of brain physiology, neuronal activity, and secretion of neurotransmitters, among others, change throughout the day, in such a way that the cerebral functions present circadian variations, dependent on the time of day, although it should be noted that they also depend on the sleep-wake cycle [27, 28]. Circadian rhythms in mammals are generated by the suprachiasmatic nucleus (SCN) of the hypothalamus, and both GABA and glutamate are intimately related to the function of this nucleus. Indeed, the photic information received by the SCN comes directly from the retina through the hypothalamic retinal tract, which releases glutamate, and indirectly through the hypothalamic geniculate tract that releases GABA and neuropeptide Y [29]; besides, GABA is one of the main neurotransmitters present in the SCN.

The variability in neuroprotection associated with the photoperiod can be explained by considering that the endogenous levels of practically any endogenous molecule present variations during the different phases of photoperiod. Diurnal variations have been reported in the circulating levels of heat shock proteins (HSPs) [30], as well as brain-derived neurotrophic factor (BDNF) and its receptors in the prefrontal cortex [31], of anandamide in cerebrospinal fluid, pons, hippocampus, and hypothalamus [32]. Our group found diurnal variations in CB1 cannabinoid receptor expression in the hippocampus [33], pons [34] and cerebral cortex [23].

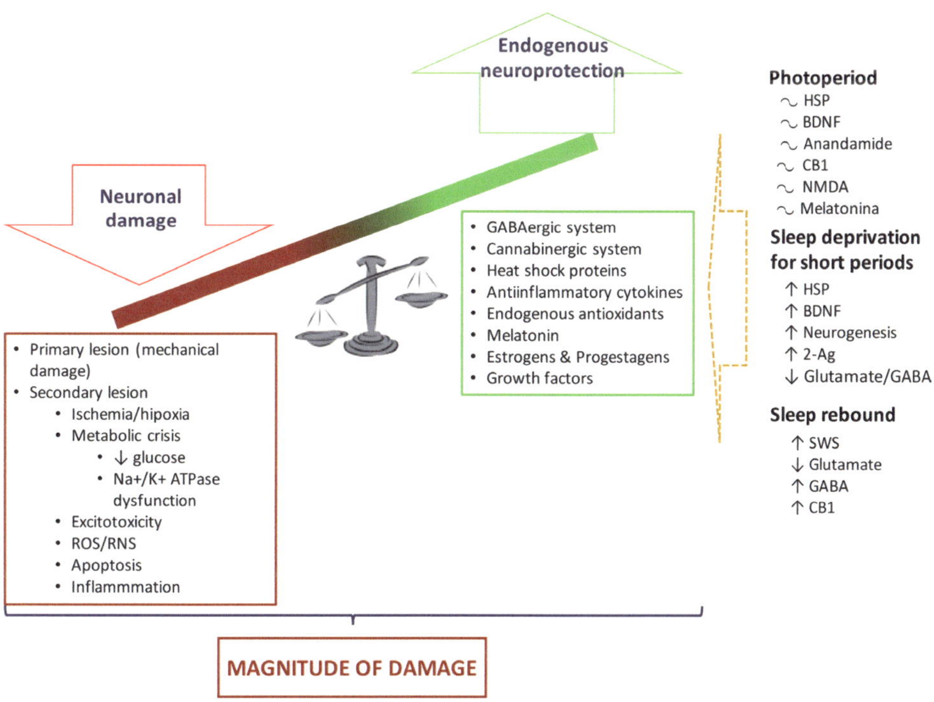

Figure 1.
Mechanisms of neuronal damage, endogenous neuroprotection, and its relationship with photoperiod, sleep deprivation for short periods, and sleep rebound. BDNF: brain-derived neurotrophic factor; CB1: cannabinoid receptor type 1; GABA: gamma-aminobutyric acid; HSP: heat shock proteins; NMDA: N-methyl-D-aspartate receptor; 2-Ag: 2-arachidonoylglycerol; and SWS: slow wave sleep. Data obtained from Refs. [4-7, 23, 24, 31-34, 71-86, 92-95].

Besides, we recently reported diurnal variations in the expression of the NMDA receptor in motor cortex [24] (see **Figure 1**).

On the other hand, it has been reported that the TBI causes circadian dysregulations of blood pressure, heart rate, body temperature [35], hormonal cycles [36], and the sleep-wake cycle [37, 38]. Patients who suffered a severe TBI do not have a perceptible sleep/wake rhythm on the first or second day after the injury, and only half of them will have recovered a consolidated day/night pattern of wakefulness and sleep, 8 days later. The recovery of a circadian organization is a predictive factor of patient wellness [39]. It has been suggested that patients with lesions in the hypothalamus and the SCN will have poor outcomes [40]. Recent data from the literature indicate that even a mild TBI causes damage in hypothalamic structural and functional connectivity [41]. Also, it has been shown that the expression of clock genes such as BMAL1 and Cry1 is disrupted in the SCN and hippocampus of rats that are subjected to TBI [42].

3. Neuroprotection and sleep

Numerous studies have documented sleep-wake disturbances (SWD) in adults post-TBI, with excessive diurnal somnolence and insomnia being the biggest complaints. However, other sleep disorders such as narcolepsy, restless leg syndrome, parasomnias, and obstructive and central sleep apnea have also been reported [39]. Several studies indicate that hypersomnia following TBI has a prevalence varying between 50 and 85% [39, 43]. If the onset of hypersomnolence is from the traumatic event, it is called posttraumatic hypersomnia (PH) and is a hallmark of severe TBI. It has been reported that PH is related to direct injury to the alerting histaminergic tuberomammillary neurons, which are reduced by approximately 40% after severe TBI [44]. Also documented are fatigue and hypersomnia following mild TBI associated with the injury of the lower portion of the ascending reticular activating system between the pontine reticular formation and the intralaminar thalamic nucleus, using diffusion tensor tractography [45].

Botchway et al. [46] reported that even 20 years after a TBI in childhood, young adulthood present increased risk of SWD and that this is more common after a moderate TBI than after a severe one.

Haboubi et al. [47] found that up to 46% of patients reported insomnia that persisted beyond 6 months after mild TBI. Insomnia is reported more frequently with milder forms of TBI injuries [48] and has been associated with head trauma involving lower frontal and anterior temporal regions, including the basal forebrain as it affects the area involved in sleep initiation [39, 49].

Zhou [41], using advanced quantitative magnetic resonance imaging techniques, showed that disruption of functional and structural hypothalamic connectivity in patients with mild TBI was associated with fatigue and sleep problems.

Hypersomnolence has been associated with a decrease in the number of hypocretin-positive cells in experimental TBI models [50–52]. Also, an increased number of awakenings associated with an increase in reactive microglia in thalamic regions have been reported [53].

On the other hand, there are few data in the literature that support the neuroprotective role of sleep or wakefulness. Although, when a child falls and hits his/her head, a general recommendation says: "Do not let him sleep"; there is no reliable data in the literature to support that this sleep deprivation will have some protective effect. More informed recommendations indicate that if the child is sleepy, he/she is allowed to sleep, but that he must be awakened every 2 h to verify that he/she speaks, moves the four extremities and that is oriented [54].

It is worth noting that there is extensive literature that supports that sleep deprivation for prolonged periods impairs many physiological functions and causes death [55–58]. Total sleep deprivation (TSD) in rats causes deterioration in health whose end is death in a period between 11 and 32 days [56], while selectively rapid eye movement sleep deprivation (REMSD) causes death between 16 and 54 days [57].

Nevertheless, recent evidence suggests that sleep deprivation for shorter periods may be neuroprotective. Indeed, several studies in focal and global cerebral ischemia [59, 61, 65–67], cardiac arrest [60] or TBI [64, 68, 69] murine models have documented that both TSD [59, 61, 64–66, 69] and REMSD [60, 64, 67] have neuroprotective effects, whether they are applied before the insult [59–61, 65, 66] or after it [64, 67, 69] as summarized in **Table 1**. However, some studies indicate that sleep deprivation for short periods had no effect [68] or, its effect was deleterious [62, 63] (see **Table 1**).

As can be seen in **Table 1**, in some of the cases, sleep deprivation for short periods of time was applied before the noxious stimulus so it could be considered as a preconditioning stimulus [70], that is, a stimulus that triggers the activation of the endogenous neuroprotection response and prepares the organism against a harmful event of greater wingspan. However, in other studies indicated in **Table 1**, sleep deprivation for short periods was applied after the noxious stimulus, so it would rather act as a neuroprotective factor by delaying and/or decreasing the secondary lesion. In this sense, several reports in the literature suggest that sleep deprivation for short periods increase the expression of neuroprotective molecules like HSP, growth factors, and plasticity-related genes [71–73]. It also has been reported that TSD for short periods produces neurogenesis in the hippocampus [74, 75] (see **Figure 1**).

Another factor that could be participating in the neuroprotective role of sleep deprivation for short periods is the balance between glutamatergic and GABAergic systems, which both sleep deprivation and TBI produce. In the literature, there are reports that TBI increases both glutamate [76–78] and GABA [79]. Also, the expression of GABAA receptors [80, 81] and NMDA [82] is modified; there are also several reports that indicate that sleep deprivation for short periods changes the release of both glutamate and GABA. REMSD increases the level of glutamate [83], as well as that of GABA but reduces the glutamate/GABA ratio [84]. These modifications could be significant in events such as TBI or ischemia since they would be regulating the excitotoxicity produced by glutamate. They could also be correlated with reports showing that sleep deprivation for short periods modifies the expression and/or replacement of NMDA receptors [85, 86]. For example, McDermott [87] shows that the REMSD for 72 h increases the intracellular NMDA levels, which could be interpreted as a down-regulation in response to the increase of glutamate; in the same way, several investigations show that the sleep deprivation for short periods can be an event that prevents the glutamate toxicity mediated by NMDA receptors [88]. As for GABAA receptors, there are reports that sleep deprivation for short periods increases their expression [89, 90], and/or modifies the expression of some subunits, which may explain functional changes in GABAergic transmission [91].

The cannabinergic system could also be participating in the neuroprotective effect of sleep deprivation for short periods. It has been reported that circulating 2-Ag increases with sleep deprivation [92].

Also, it is worth noting that TSD induces a subsequent increase or rebound in slow-wave or high-amplitude electroencephalographic activity during slow wave sleep (SWS) while REMD induces an increase or rebound in REMS [93], so it is possible that the sleep rebound is the neuroprotective factor. This is in agreement with the findings of Brager et al. [94] who utilized remote preconditioning to prevent damage in a focal brain ischemia model. They found that remote preconditioning was associated with an increase of SWS. Also, sleep rebound appears to reduce the cerebral cortex level of glutamate [83] and increase that of GABA [95]. Besides, we have documented that the rebound after REMSD increases the expression of the CB1 cannabinoid receptors in the rat pons [34], which could have a neuroprotective effect.

Also, during sleep rebound, the function of the glymphatic system is favored and therefore the elimination of toxic brain substances [96–98].

Reference	Damage model	Sleep deprivation (method and schedule)	Main findings	Outcome
Hsu et al. [59]	Global cerebral ischemia in rat	TSD for 5 days before a transient global cerebral ischemia	Attenuation of the damage of pyramidal cells in the hippocampal CA1 and glial reactions	⇑
Weil et al. [60]	Cardiac arrest in mice	48 h of REMSD immediately before cardiac arrest	Improved ischemic outcome. Lesser neuronal hippocampal damage and increased gene expression of IL-6 and IL-10	⇑
Moldovan et al. [61]	Focal cerebral ischemia in rat	6 h of TSD immediately before focal cerebral ischemia	Decreased loss of functions and a smaller infarct volume	⇑
Gao et al. [62]	Focal cerebral ischemia in rat	TSD for 12 h, 12 h after focal cerebral ischemia. TSD for 12 h, for consecutive 3 days 12 h after ischemia	Both sleep deprivation schedules increased the infarct volume and the number of damaged cells	⇓
Zunzunegui et al. [63]	Focal cerebral ischemia in rat	TSD for 12 h, for consecutive 3 days 12 h after ischemia	Lower recovery of forearm motor skills, reduction in axonal sprouting, and synaptophysin expression	⇓
Martinez Vargas et al. [64]	TBI in rat	REMSD and TSD for 24 h immediately after a moderate TBI	Increase in the neurobehavioral recovery and reduction in the histological damage	⇑
Cam et al. [65]	Focal cerebral ischemia in rat	6 h of TSD immediately before focal cerebral ischemia	Reduction in infarct volume associated with an increase in the amount of SWS and REMS.	⇑
Pace et al. [66]	Focal cerebral ischemia in rat	6 h of TSD immediately before focal cerebral ischemia	Reduction in infarct volume associated with a reduction in up-regulation of genes involved in cell cycle regulation and immune response.	⇑
Cheng et al. [67]	Global cerebral ischemia in rat	REMSD for 12 h/day for 3 days 48 h after global cerebral ischemia and reperfusion	Improvement in cognitive function, increased number of BrdU- and BrdU/NSE-positive cells as well as hippocampal BDNF expression	⇑
Caron and Stephenson [68]	TBI in rat	TSD for 48 h or chronic sleep restriction (6 h of sleep/day for 10 days) following mild TBI	TSD or CSR did not exacerbate the neuronal damage induced by TBI	=
Morawska et al. [69]	TBI in rat	Increased sleep with sodium oxybate or TSD (6 h daily/5 d) starting 1 day after TBI	Enhanced encephalographic slow-wave activity. Markedly reduced diffuse axonal damage in the cortex and hippocampus, and improved memory impairment	⇑

SWS, slow wave sleep; REMS, rapid eye movement sleep; TBI, traumatic brain injury; and CSR, Chronic sleep restriction.

Table 1.
REMSD, rapid eye movement sleep deprivation. TSD, total sleep deprivation.

4. Sleep deprivation in humans

The TSD or REMSD data for short periods indicated in the previous section were obtained in animal models, but what is known in humans?

Recent studies indicate that our society is sleeping less and less and that this has a negative impact on health and wellbeing. Between 7 and 8 h/night of sleep is recommended in adults, although this time varies from person to person. Having an insufficient sleep in quantity or quality for multiple nights causes a debt of sleep that cannot be recovered and increases the risk of stroke, obesity, diabetes Mellitus type 2, and cardiovascular disease [99].

However, numerous studies have reported the effectiveness of TSD for one night in patients with depression; the first to report this were Pflug and Tolle, in 1971 [100]. Subsequently, Vogel et al. [101] described that the REMSD was also effective. Gillin [102], in 1983, pointed out that of a total of 852 patients who were TSD or REMSD for one or more nights, 493 (57.9%) were reported to have "improved", but it is recognized that this improvement in mood is transient and it is currently recommended that the TSD or REMSD be combined with sleep phase advance (SPA), pharmacotherapy, and sometimes also phototherapy [103].

Several studies have tried to find the mechanism by which the TSD or REMSD are effective in mood improvement. In this sense, some of the effects of sleep deprivation or the rebound could be considered as neuroprotective; for example, Davies et al. observed that TSD for 24 h increases the serum levels of tryptophan, taurine, and serotonin, which could explain, in part, the antidepressant effect of deprivation [104]. It is worth noting that taurine has been related to cell volume changes triggered by different neurological diseases that produce secondary damage to ischemia [105]. This role is associated with its participation as osmolyte, which has been demonstrated by characterizing the increase in its extracellular concentration and its decrease in the intracellular one. Taurine can regulate the edema induced by the glutamate released during the excitotoxic cascade after a TBI. The nonvesicular release of taurine is an essential protective mechanism to prevent cell lysis, since, upon release to the extracellular environment, there is a change in the direction of mobilization of ions and water [106].

Hefti et al. [107] showed an increased expression of mGluR5 glutamate receptor in the cingulate cortex, insula, medial temporal lobe, parahippocampal gyrus, striatum, and amygdala of healthy men after 33 h of TSD. Previously, some authors had reported that the activation of this receptor decreases the damage, using animal models of cerebral focal ischemia [108] and spinal cord injury [109].

Gorgulu and Caliyurt [110] demonstrated an increase in the concentration of serum BDNF in patients with depression treated with three overnight TSD over a week; nevertheless, in healthy subjects, TSD did not affect the level of BDNF.

In the course of TSD, the concentration of cortisol increases considerably as a result of stimulation of the hypothalamic-pituitary-adrenal axis. The rebound after TSD resulted in a significant reduction of cortisol and increase of growth hormone (GH) secretion driven by the increase of SWS [111]. Recently, neuroprotection has been identified as one of the functions of GH [112, 113].

Also, the level of thyroid hormones increases during sleep deprivation. It is the result of the stimulation of the hypothalamic-pituitary-thyroid axis [114]. It has also been described that thyroid hormones play a neuroprotective role in acute cerebrovascular disorders [115].

However, some studies show effects of TSD that could not be considered as neuroprotective; for example, Trivedi et al. [116] found that glutathione, ATP, cysteine, and homocysteine levels in plasma were significantly reduced as a result of one night of TSD, while Meier-Ewert et al. [117] reported that one night of TSD increased serum C reactive protein concentrations. Also, one night of TSD causes an increase of serum concentration of interleukin 6 (IL-6), a proinflammatory cytokine in depressive patients as in healthy subjects; but in healthy individuals sleep rebound increased the level of interleukin-1-receptor antagonist (IL-1RA) [118], which inhibits the action of the proinflammatory interleukins 1alpha and 1beta.

Some deleterious effects attributed to the TSD may be influenced by the deprivation method; for example, Gil-Lozano et al. [119] reported that overnight TSD with nocturnal light exposure disrupted the melatonin and cortisol profiles and increased insulin resistance. These alterations were not observed in TSD participants maintained under dark conditions.

5. Limitations

Studies on the impact of acute sleep deprivation and its neuroprotective effects in humans against acquired brain damage are scarce. However, studies performed in subjects without brain injury indicate the existence of neuroprotective mechanisms, as long as it is a TSD for short or acute periods (24 h). In order to propose sleep deprivation as a neuroprotective mechanism and incorporate it as part of the treatment against TBI, more studies are still needed.

6. Perspectives

The importance of the TBI as a public health problem worldwide requires us to understand the pathophysiological changes underlying this neurological event, as well as the processes that favor the activation of endogenous neuroprotection, in order to apply them as a possible therapeutic strategy.

The previous evidence highlights the importance of considering the time of the day when acquired brain injury is established. The alterations found as a consequence of this event are heterogeneous and complex, ranging from molecular changes to behavioral modifications; as pointed before, TBI causes dysregulation of sleep-wake cycle and homeostasis unbalance including many neuropeptide and hormones changes.

In many of the alterations induced by an acquired brain damage, the participation of neurotransmission systems such as GABAergic, glutamatergic, and cannabinergic is fundamental. These, like all endogenous molecules, have a diurnal variation; such variations, in the same way, affect the sleep-wake cycle. Evidence in animal models of the neuroprotective effect of sleep deprivation for short periods encourages us to continue researching this.

Knowing the relationship between neuroprotection, photoperiod, and sleep, as well as the participation of the neurotransmission systems involved in the TBI, opens a window in their study as potential biomarkers or therapeutic targets. With this approach, it will probably benefit a higher number of patients with acquired brain damage.

Acknowledgements

This work was supported by PAPIIT IN223417.

Author details

Marina Martinez-Vargas, Mercedes Graciela Porras-Villalobos, Francisco Estrada-Rojo, Ricardo Jesus Martinez-Tapia, Adan Perez-Arredondo, Antonio Barajas-Martinez and Luz Navarro*
Department of Physiology, Faculty of Medicine, National Autonomous University of Mexico, Cd. Mx., Mexico

*Address all correspondence to: lnavarro@unam.mx

References

[1] LetechipIa-Vallejo G, Morali de la Brena G, Cervantes-Alfaro JM. Neuroprotección. Neuroprotectores endogenos. In: Velazquez-Moctezuma J, editor. Temas Selectos de Neurociencias. Mexico D.F.: UAM; 2004. pp. 159-168

[2] Leonard AL. History of neuroprotection and rationale as a therapy for glaucoma. The American Journal of Managed Care. 2008;**14**:S11-S14

[3] Jain KK. Handbook of Neuroprotection. Basel: Humana Press; 2011. p. 1

[4] Leker RR, Shohami E. Cerebral ischemia and trauma-different etiologies yet similar mechanisms: Neuroprotective opportunities. Brain Research Reviews. 2002;**39**:55-73

[5] Nestler EJ et al. Seizures and stroke. In: Molecular Neuropharmacology. A Foundation for Clinical Neuroscience. NY: McGraw-Hill; 2000. pp. 479-503

[6] Lee JM, Grabb MC, Zipfel GJ, Choi DW. Brain tissue responses to ischemia. The Journal of Clinical Investigation. 2000;**106**(6):723-731

[7] Shohami E, Cohen-Yeshurun A, Magid L, Algali M, Mechoulam R. Endocannabinoids and traumatic brain injury. British Journal of Pharmacology. 2011;**163**(7):1402-1410. DOI: 10.1111/j.1476-5381.2011.01343.x

[8] Lyden PD. GABA and neuroprotection. International Review of Neurobiology. 1997;**40**:233-258

[9] Grewer C, Gameiro A, Zhang Z, Tao Z, Braams S, Rauen T. Glutamate forward and reverse transport: From molecular mechanism to transporter-mediated release after ischemia. IUBMB Life. 2008;**60**(9):609-619. DOI: 10.1002/iub.98

[10] Gouix E, Lèveillè F, Nicole O, Melon C, Had-Aissouni L, Buisson A. Reverse glial glutamate uptake triggers neuronal cell death through extrasynaptic NMDA receptor activation. Molecular and Cellular Neurosciences. 2009;**40**(4):463-473

[11] Zoghbi HY et al. Neurobiology of disease. Current Opinion in Neurobiology. 2000;**10**:655-660

[12] OíDell DM et al. Positive and negative modulation of the GABA receptor and outcome after a traumatic brain injury in rats. Brain Research. 2000;**861**:325-332

[13] Xu J et al. Additive neuroprotection of GABA A and GABA B receptor agonists in cerebral ischemic injury via PI-3K/Akt pathway inhibiting the ASK1-JNK cascade. Neuropharmacology. 2008;**54**:1029-1040

[14] Panikashvili D, Simeonidou C, Ben-Shabat S, Hanus L, Breuer A, Mechoulam R, et al. An endogenous cannabinoid (2-AG) is neuroprotective after brain injury. Nature. 2001;**413**:527-531

[15] Mechoulam R, Spatz M, Shohami E. Endocannabinoids and neuroprotection. Science's STKE. 2002;**2002**(129):re5

[16] Mechoulam R. Discovery of endocannabinoids and some random thoughts on their possible roles in neuroprotection and aggression. Prostaglandins, Leukotrienes and Essential FattyAcids. 2002;**66**(2&3):93-99

[17] Xu JY, Chen C. Endocannabinoids in synaptic plasticity and neuroprotection. The Neuroscientist. 2015;**21**(2):152-168. DOI: 10.1177/1073858414524632

[18] Marler J. Circadian variation in stroke onset. In: Deedwania PC, editor.

Circadian Rhythms of Cardiovascular Disorders. Armonk, NY: Futura Publishing Co Inc.; 1993. pp. 163-172

[19] Chaturvedi S, Adams HP Jr, Woolson RF. Circadian variation in ischemic stroke subtypes. Stroke. 1999;**30**(9):1792-1795

[20] Raj K, Bhatia R, Prasad K, Srivastava MV, Vishnubhatla S, Singh MB. Seasonal differences and circadian variation in stroke occurrence and stroke subtypes. Journal of Stroke and Cerebrovascular Diseases. 2015;**24**(1):10-16. DOI: 10.1016/j.jstrokecerebrovasdis.2014.07.051

[21] Vinall PE, Kramer MS, Heinel LA, Rosenwasser RH. Temporal changes in sensitivity of rats to cerebral ischemic insult. Journal of Neurosurgery. 2000;**93**:82-89

[22] Martinez-Vargas M, Gonzalez-Rivera R, Soto-Nuñez M, Cisneros-Martinez M, Huerta-Saquero A, Morales-Gomez J, et al. Recovery after a traumatic brain injury depends on diurnal variations. Effect of cystatin C. Neuroscience Letters. 2006;**400**:21-24

[23] Martinez-Vargas M, Morales-Gomez J, Gonzalez-Rivera R, Hernandez-Enriquez C, Perez-Arredondo A, Estrada-Rojo F, et al. Does the neuroprotective role of anandamide display diurnal variations? International Journal of Molecular Sciences. 2013;**14**(12):23341-23355. DOI: 10.3390/ijms141223341

[24] Estrada-Rojo F, Morales-Gomez J, Coballase-Urrutia E, Martinez-Vargas M, Navarro L. Diurnal variation of NMDA receptor expression in the rat cerebral cortex is associated with traumatic brain injury damage. BMC Research Notes. 2018;**11**(1):150. DOI: 10.1186/s13104-018-3258-0

[25] Gruart A, Delgado JM, Escobar C, Aguilar-Roblero R. Los relojes que gobiernan la vida. In: La ciencia para todos 188. México, D.F.: Fondo de Cultura Economica; 2002

[26] Jagannath A, Taylor L, Wakaf Z, Vasudevan SR, Foster RG. The genetics of circadian rhythms, sleep, and health. Human Molecular Genetics. 2017;**26**(R2):R128-R138. DOI: 10.1093/hmg/ddx240

[27] Valdez P, Ramirez C, Garcia A, Talamantes J. Los cambios en la atención a lo largo del día. Ciencia. 2008;**59**:14-23

[28] Leproult R, Persson PB. Enhanced mental performance at higher body temperature? American Journal of Physiology. Regulatory, Integrative and Comparative Physiology. 2002;**283**:R1368-R1369

[29] Akiyama M, Moriya T, Shibata S. Physiological, pharmacological and molecular aspects of mammalian biological clocks. Nippon Yakurigaku Zasshi. 1998;**112**:243-250

[30] Sandström ME, Madden LA, Taylor L, Siegler JC, Lovell RJ, Midgley A, et al. Variation in basal heat shock protein 70 is correlated to core temperature in human subjects. Amino Acids. 2009;**37**(2):279-284. DOI: 10.1007/s00726-008-0144-4

[31] Coria-Lucero CD, Golini RS, Ponce IT, Deyurka N, Anzulovich AC, Delgado SM, et al. Rhythmic BDNF and TrkB expression patterns in the prefrontal cortex are lost in aged rats. Brain Research. 2016;**1653**:51-58. DOI: 10.1016/j.brainres.2016.10.019

[32] Murillo-Rodriguez E, Desarnaud F, Prospero-Garcia O. Diurnal variation of arachidonoylethanolamine, palmitoylethanolamide and oleoylethanolamide in the brain of the rat. Life Sciences. 2006;**79**(1):30-37

[33] Rueda-Orozco PE, Soria-Gomez E, Montes-Rodriguez CJ, Martinez-Vargas M, Galicia O, Navarro L, et al. A potential

function of endocannabinoids in the selection of a navigation strategy by rats. Psychopharmacology. 2008;**198**(4):565-576

[34] Martínez-Vargas M, Murillo-Rodríguez E, Gonz·lez-Rivera R, Landa A, Méndez-Diaz M, Prospero-García O, et al. Sleep modulates cannabinoid receptor 1 expression in the pons of rats. Neuroscience. 2003;**117**(1):197-201

[35] Paul T, Lemmer B. Disturbance of circadian rhythms in analgosedated intensive care unit patients with and without craniocerebral injury. Chronobiology International. 2007;**24**:45-61

[36] Llompart-Pou J, Perez G, Raurich JM, Riesco M, Brell M, IbaÒez J, et al. Loss of cortisol circadian rhythm in patients with traumatic brain injury: A microdialysis evaluation. Neurocritical Care. 2010;**13**:211-216

[37] Ayalon L, Borodkin K, Dishon L, Kanety H, Dagan Y. Circadian rhythm sleep disorders following mild traumatic brain injury. Neurology. 2007;**8**:1136-1140

[38] Castriotta RJ, Murthy JN. Sleep disorders in patients with traumatic brain injury: A review. CNS Drugs. 2010;**25**:175-185

[39] Wolfe LF, Sahni AS, Attarian H. Sleep disorders in traumatic brain injury. NeuroRehabilitation. 2018;**43**(3):257-266. DOI: 10.3233/NRE-182583

[40] Duclos C, Dumont M, Blais H, Paquet J, Laflamme E, de Beaumont L, et al. Rest-activity cycle disturbances in the acute phase of moderate to severe traumatic brain injury. Neurorehabilitation and Neural Repair. 2014;**28**(5):472-482. DOI: 10.1177/1545968313517756

[41] Zhou Y. Abnormal structural and functional hypothalamic connectivity in mild traumatic brain injury. Journal of Magnetic Resonance Imaging. 2017;**45**(4):1105-1112. DOI: 10.1002/jmri.25413

[42] Boone DR, Sell SL, Micci MA, Crookshanks JM, Parsley M, Uchida T, et al. Traumatic brain injury-induced dysregulation of the circadian clock. PLoS One. 2012;**7**:e46204

[43] Mathias JL, Alvaro PK. Prevalence of sleep disturbances, disorders, and problems following traumatic brain injury: A meta-analysis. Sleep Medicine. 2012;**13**(7):898-905. DOI: 10.1016/j.sleep.2012.04.006

[44] Valko PO, Gavrilov YV, Yamamoto M, Finn K, Reddy H, Haybaeck J, et al. Damage to histaminergic tuberomammillary neurons and other hypothalamic neurons with traumatic brain injury. Annals of Neurology. 2015;**77**(1):177-182. DOI: 10.1002/ana.24298

[45] Jang SH, Kwon HG. Injury of the ascending reticular activating system in patients with fatigue and hypersomnia following mild traumatic brain injury: Two case reports. Medicine (Baltimore). 2016;**95**(6):e2628. DOI: 10.1097/MD.0000000000002628

[46] Botchway EN, Godfrey C, Anderson V, Nicholas CL, Catroppa C. Outcomes of subjective sleep-wake disturbances twenty years after traumatic brain injury in childhood. Journal of Neurotrauma. 2019;**36**(5):669-678. DOI: 10.1089/neu.2018.5743

[47] Haboubi NH, Long J, Koshy M, Ward AB. Short-term sequelae of minor head injury (6 years experience of minor head injury clinic). Disability and Rehabilitation. 2001;**23**(14):635-638

[48] Kaufman Y, Tzischinsky O, Epstein R, Etzioni A, Lavie P, Pillar G.

Long-term sleep disturbances in adolescents after minor head injury. Pediatric Neurology. 2001;**24**(2):129-134

[49] Viola-Saltzman M, Watson NF. Traumatic brain injury and sleep disorders. Neurologic Clinics. 2012;**30**(4):1299-1312. DOI: 10.1016/j.ncl.2012.08.008

[50] Rowe RK, Harrison JL, Morrison H, Subbian V, Murphy SM, Lifshitz J. Acute post-traumatic sleep may define vulnerability to a second traumatic brain injury in mice. Journal of Neurotrauma. 18 Dec 2018. DOI: 10.1089/neu.2018.5980

[51] Skopin MD, Kabadi SV, Viechweg SS, Mong JA, Faden AI. Chronic decrease in wakefulness and disruption of sleep-wake behavior after experimental traumatic brain injury. Journal of Neurotrauma. 2015;**32**(5):289-296. DOI: 10.1089/neu.2014.3664

[52] Thomasy HE, Opp MR. Hypocretin mediates sleep and wake disturbances in a mouse model of traumatic brain injury. Journal of Neurotrauma. 2019;**36**(5):802-814. DOI: 10.1089/neu.2018.5810

[53] Hazra A, Macolino C, Elliott MB, Chin J. Delayed thalamic astrocytosis and disrupted sleep-wake patterns in a preclinical model of traumatic brain injury. Journal of Neuroscience Research. 2014;**92**(11):1434-1445. DOI: 10.1002/jnr.23430

[54] Gudeman SK. Textbook of Head Injury. Philadelphia: Saunders; 1989

[55] Barriga C, Rodriguez A, Esteban S, Rial R. Interrelations between sleep and the immune status. Revista de Neurologia. 2005;**40**:548-556

[56] Everson CA, Bergmann BB, Rechtschaffen A. Sleep deprivation in the rat: III. Total sleep deprivation. Sleep. 1989;**12**:13-21

[57] Kushida CA, Bergmann BM, Rechtschaffen A. Sleep deprivation in the rat: IV. Paradoxical sleep deprivation. Sleep. 1989;**12**:22-30

[58] Rechtschaffen A, Gilliland MA, Bergmann BM, Winter JB. Physiological correlates of prolonged sleep deprivation in rats. Science. 1983;**221**:182-184

[59] Hsu JC, Lee YS, Chang CN, Ling EA, Lan CT. Sleep deprivation prior to transient global cerebral ischemia attenuates glial reaction in the rat hippocampal formation. Brain Research. 2003;**984**:170-181

[60] Weil ZM, Norman GJ, Karelina K, Morris JS, Barker JM, Su AJ, et al. Sleep deprivation attenuates inflammatory responses and ischemic cell death. Experimental Neurology. 2009;**218**:129-136

[61] Moldovan M, Constantinescu AO, Balseanu A, Oprescu N, Zagrean L, Popa-Wagner A. Sleep deprivation attenuates experimental stroke severity in rats. Experimental Neurology. 2010;**222**:135-143

[62] Gao B, Cam E, Jaeger H, Zunzunegui C, Sarnthein J, Bassetti CL. Sleep disruption aggravates focal cerebral ischemia in the rat. Sleep. 2010;**33**:879-887

[63] Zunzunegui C, Gao B, Cam E, Hodor A, Bassetti CL. Sleep disturbance impairs stroke recovery in the rat. Sleep. 2011;**34**:1261-1269

[64] Martinez-Vargas M, Estrada Rojo F, Tabla-Ramon E, Navarro-Arguelles H, Ortiz-Lailzon N, Hernandez-Chavez A, et al. Sleep deprivation has a neuroprotective role in a traumatic brain injury of the rat. Neuroscience Letters. 2012;**529**(2):118-122. DOI: 10.1016/j.neulet.2012.09.037

[65] Cam E, Gao B, Imbach L, Hodor A, Bassetti CL. Sleep deprivation

before stroke is neuroprotective: A pre-ischemic conditioning related to sleep rebound. Experimental Neurology. 2013;**247**:673-679. DOI: 10.1016/j.expneurol.2013.03.003

[66] Pace M, Baracchi F, Gao B, Bassetti C. Identification of sleep-modulated pathways involved in neuroprotection from stroke. Sleep. 2015;**38**(11):1707-1718. DOI: 10.5665/sleep.5148

[67] Cheng O, Li R, Zhao L, Yu L, Yang B, Wang J, et al. Short-term sleep deprivation stimulates hippocampal neurogenesis in rats following global cerebral ischemia/reperfusion. PLoS One. 2015;**10**(6):e0125877. DOI: 10.1371/journal.pone.0125877

[68] Caron AM, Stephenson R. Sleep deprivation does not affect neuronal susceptibility to mild traumatic brain injury in the rat. Nature and Science of Sleep. 2015;7:63-72. DOI: 10.2147/NSS.S82888

[69] Morawska MM, Büchele F, Moreira CG, Imbach LL, Noain D, Baumann CR. Sleep modulation alleviates axonal damage and cognitive decline after rodent traumatic brain injury. The Journal of Neuroscience. 2016;**36**(12):3422-3429. DOI: 10.1523/JNEUROSCI.3274-15.2016

[70] Pincherle A, Pace M, Sarasso S, Facchin L, Dreier JP, Bassetti CL. Sleep, preconditioning and stroke. Stroke. 2017;**48**(12):3400-3407. DOI: 10.1161/STROKEAHA.117.018796

[71] Tononi G, Cirelli C. Modulation of brain gene expression during sleep and wakefulness: A review of recent findings. Neuropsychopharmacology. 2001;**25**(Suppl):S28-S35

[72] Cirelli C, Gutierrez CM, Tononi G. Extensive and divergent effects of sleep and wakefulness on brain gene expression. Neuron. 2004;**41**(1):35-43

[73] Elliott AS, Huber JD, OíCallaghan JP, Rosen CL, Miller DB. A review of sleep deprivation studies the brain transcriptome. Springerplus. 2014;**3**:728

[74] Grassi Zucconi G, Cipriani S, Balgkouranidou I, Scattoni R. One night sleep deprivation stimulates hippocampal neurogenesis. Brain Research Bulletin. 2006;**69**:375-381

[75] Junek A, Rusak B, Semba K. Short-term sleep deprivation may alter the dynamics of hippocampal cell proliferation in adult rats. Neuroscience. 2010;**170**:1140-1152

[76] Faden AI, Demediuk P, Panter SS, Vink R. The role of excitatory amino acids and NMDA receptors in traumatic brain injury. Science. 1989;**244**(4906):798-800

[77] Katayama Y, Becker DP, Tamura T, Hovda DA. Massive increases in extracellular potassium and the indiscriminate release of glutamate following concussive brain injury. Journal of Neurosurgery. 1990 Dec;**73**(6):889-900

[78] Globus MY, Alonso O, Dietrich WD, Busto R, Ginsberg MD. Glutamate release and free radical production following brain injury: Effects of posttraumatic hypothermia. Journal of Neurochemistry. 1995;**65**(4):1704-1711

[79] Zhong C et al. NAAG peptidase inhibitor increases dialysate NAAG and reduces glutamate, aspartate and GABA levels in the dorsal hippocampus following fluid percussion injury in the rat. Journal of Neurochemistry. 2006;**97**(4):1015-1025

[80] Neumann-Haefelin T et al. Upregulation of GABA-receptor a1- and a2-subunit mRNAs following a ischemic cortical lesions in rats. Brain Research. 1999;**816**:234-237

[81] Mtchedlishvili Z, Lepsveridze E, Xu H, Kharlamov EA, Lu B, Kelly KM.

Increase of GABAA receptor-mediated tonic inhibition in dentate granule cells after traumatic brain injury. Neurobiology of Disease. 2010;**38**(3):464-475. DOI: 10.1016/j.nbd.2010.03.012

[82] Kumar A, Zou L, Yuan X, Long Y, Yang K. N-methyl-D-aspartate receptors: Transient loss of NR1/NR2A/NR2B subunits after traumatic brain injury in a rodent model. Journal of Neuroscience Research. 2002;**67**(6):781-786

[83] Dash MB, Douglas CL, Vyazovskiy VV, Cirelli C, Tononi G. Long-term homeostasis of extracellular glutamate in the rat cerebral cortex across sleep and waking states. The Journal of Neuroscience. 2009;**29**(3):620-629. DOI: 10.1523/JNEUROSCI.5486-08.2009

[84] Wang SX, Li QS. Effects of sleep deprivation on gamma-amino-butyric acid and glutamate contents in rat brain. Di Yi Jun Yi Da Xue Xue Bao. 2002;**22**(10):888-890

[85] Longordo F et al. Consequences of sleep deprivation on neurotransmitter receptor expression and function. The European Journal of Neuroscience. 2009;**29**(9):1810-1819

[86] Longordo F et al. NR2A at CA1 synapses is obligatory for the susceptibility of hippocampal plasticity to sleep loss. The Journal of Neuroscience. 2009;**29**(28):9026-9041

[87] McDermott CM et al. Sleep deprivation-induced alterations in excitatory synaptic transmission in the CA1 region of the rat hippocampus. The Journal of Physiology. 2006;**570** (Pt 3):553-565

[88] Novati A, Hulshof HJ, Granic I, Meerlo P. Chronic partial sleep deprivation reduces brain sensitivity to glutamate N-methyl-D-aspartate receptor-mediated neurotoxicity. Journal of Sleep Research. 2012;**21**(1):3-9. DOI: 10.1111/j.1365-2869.2011.00932.x

[89] Pokk P et al. Is upregulation of benzodiazepine receptors a compensatory reaction to reduced GABAergic tone in the brain of stressed mice? Naunyn-Schmiedeberg's Archives of Pharmacology. 1996;**354**(6):703-708

[90] Cirelli C, Tononi G. Gene expression in the brain across the sleep-waking cycle. Brain Research. 2000;**885**(2):303-321

[91] Modirrousta M, Mainville L, Jones BE. Dynamic changes in GABAA receptors on basal forebrain cholinergic neurons following sleep deprivation and recovery. BMC Neuroscience. 2007;**8**:15

[92] Hanlon EC, Tasali E, Leproult R, Stuhr KL, Doncheck E, de Wit H, et al. Sleep restriction enhances the daily rhythm of circulating levels of endocannabinoid 2-arachidonoylglycerol. Sleep. 2016;**39**(3):653-664. DOI: 10.5665/sleep.5546

[93] Rechtschaffen A, Bergmann BM, Gilliland MA, Bauer K. Effects of method, duration, and sleep stage on rebounds from sleep deprivation in the rat. Sleep. 1999;**22**(1):11-31

[94] Brager AJ, Yang T, Ehlen JC, Simon RP, Meller R, Paul KN. Sleep is critical for remote preconditioning-induced neuroprotection. Sleep. 2016;**39**(11):2033-2040

[95] Bettendorff L et al. Paradoxical sleep deprivation increases the content of glutamate and glutamine in rat cerebral cortex. Sleep. 1996;**19**(1):65-71

[96] Jessen NA, Munk AS, Lundgaard I, Nedergaard M. The glymphatic system: A Beginner's guide. Neurochemical Research. 2015;**40**(12):2583-2599. DOI: 10.1007/s11064-015-1581-6

[97] Rasmussen MK, Mestre H, Nedergaard M. The glymphatic pathway in neurological disorders. Lancet Neurology. 2018;**17**(11):1016-1024. 10.1016/S1474-4422(18)30318-1

[98] Eugene AR, Masiak J. The neuroprotective aspects of sleep. MEDtube Science. 2015;**3**(1):35-40

[99] Abrams RM. Sleep deprivation. Obstetrics and Gynecology Clinics of North America. 2015;**42**(3):493-506. DOI: 10.1016/j.ogc.2015.05.013

[100] Pflug B, Tőlle R. Therapie endogener depressionen durch schlafentzug. Nervenarzt. 1971;**42**:117-124

[101] Vogel GW, Vogel F, McAbee RS, Thurmond AJ. Improvement of depression by REM sleep deprivation, new findings and a theory. Archives of General Psychiatry. 1980;**37**:247-253

[102] Gillin JC. The sleep therapies of depression. Progress in Neuro-Psychopharmacology & Biological Psychiatry. 1983;**7**:351-364

[103] Dopierała E, Rybakowski J. Sleep deprivation as a method of chronotherapy in the treatment of depression. Psychiatria Polska. 2015;**49**(3):423-433. DOI: 10.12740/PP/30455

[104] Davies SK, Ang JE, Revell VL, Holmes B, Mann A, Robertson FP, et al. Effect of sleep deprivation on the human metabolome. Proceedings of the National Academy of Sciences of the United States of America. 2014;**111**(29):10761-10766. DOI: 10.1073/pnas.1402663111

[105] Nilsson P, Hillered L, Pontén U, Ungerstedt U. Changes in cortical extracellular levels of energy-related metabolites and amino acids following concussive brain injury in rats. Journal of Cerebral Blood Flow and Metabolism. 1990;**10**(5):631-637

[106] Stover JF, Unterberg AW. Increased cerebrospinal fluid glutamate and taurine concentrations are associated with traumatic brain edema formation in rats. Brain Research. 2000;**875**(1-2):51-55

[107] Hefti K, Holst SC, Sovago J, Bachmann V, Buck A, Ametamey SM, et al. Increased metabotropic glutamate receptor subtype 5 availability in human brain after one night without sleep. Biological Psychiatry. 2013;**73**(2):161-168. DOI: 10.1016/j.biopsych.2012.07.030

[108] Bao WL, Williams AJ, Faden AI, Tortella FC. Selective mGluR5 receptor antagonist or agonist provides neuroprotection in a rat model of focal cerebral ischemia. Brain Research. 2001;**922**(2):173-179

[109] Byrnes KR, Stoica B, Riccio A, Pajoohesh-Ganji A, Loane DJ, Faden AI. Activation of metabotropic glutamate receptor 5 improves recovery after spinal cord injury in rodents. Annals of Neurology. 2009;**66**(1):63-74. DOI: 10.1002/ana.21673

[110] Gorgulu Y, Caliyurt O. Rapid antidepressant effects of sleep deprivation therapy correlates with serum BDNF changes in major depression. Brain Research Bulletin. 2009;**80**(3):158-162

[111] Vgontzas AN, Mastorakos G, Bixler EO, Kales A, Gold PW, Chrousos GP. Sleep deprivation effects on the activity of the hypothalamic-pituitary-adrenal and growth axes: Potential clinical implications. Clinical Endocrinology. 1999;**51**(2):205-215

[112] Arce VM, Devesa P, Devesa J. Role of growth hormone (GH) in the treatment on neural diseases: From neuroprotection to neural repair. Neuroscience Research. 2013;**76**(4):179-186. DOI: 10.1016/j.neures.2013.03.014

[113] Arámburo C, Alba-Betancourt C, Luna M, Harvey S. Expression and function of growth hormone in the nervous system: A brief review. General and Comparative Endocrinology. 2014;**203**:35-42. DOI: 10.1016/j.ygcen.2014.04.035

[114] Pereira JC Jr, Andersen ML. The role of thyroid hormone in sleep deprivation. Medical Hypotheses. 2014;**82**(3):350-355

[115] Bunevicius A, Iervasi G, Bunevicius R. Neuroprotective actions of thyroid hormones and low-T3 syndrome as a biomarker in acute cerebrovascular disorders. Expert Review of Neurotherapeutics. 2015;**15**(3):315-326. DOI: 10.1586/14737175.2015.1013465

[116] Trivedi MS, Holger D, Bui AT, Craddock TJA, Tartar JL. Short-term sleep deprivation leads to decreased systemic redox metabolites and altered epigenetic status. PLoS One. 2017;**12**(7):e0181978. DOI: 10.1371/journal.pone.0181978

[117] Meier-Ewert HK, Ridker PM, Rifai N, Regan MM, Price NJ, Dinges DF, et al. Effect of sleep loss on C-reactive protein, an inflammatory marker of cardiovascular risk. Journal of the American College of Cardiology. 2004;**43**(4):678-683

[118] Voderholzer U, Fiebich BL, Dersch R, Feige B, Piosczyk H, Kopasz M, et al. Effects of sleep deprivation on nocturnal cytokine concentrations in depressed patients and healthy control subjects. The Journal of Neuropsychiatry and Clinical Neurosciences. 2012;**24**(3):354-366

[119] Gil-Lozano M, Hunter PM, Behan LA, Gladanac B, Casper RF, Brubaker PL. Short-term sleep deprivation with nocturnal light exposure alters time-dependent glucagon-like peptide-1 and insulin secretion in male volunteers. American Journal of Physiology. Endocrinology and Metabolism. 2016;**310**(1):E41-E50. DOI: 10.1152/ajpendo.00298.2015

Section 2

Imaging Diagnosis and Biomarkers

Chapter 3

Cumulative Mild Head Injury (CMHI) in Contact Sports

Kathryn Nel and Saraswathie Govender

Abstract

The effect of cumulative mild head injury (CMHI) in contact sports such as rugby union and football (soccer) is seen at all levels as more concussive injuries are reported each year globally and in South Africa. This is problematic as repeated concussions may lead to cognitive deficits in attention and poorer overall cognitive profiles both in the short and long term. The aim of this chapter is to present a brief review of research on CMHI in football and rugby and other sports (briefly) both international and South African underpinned by an overview of the anatomy and neuroanatomy of the brain to illustrate the mechanisms involved in head injuries. Risk factors for all types of MHI are also given.

Keywords: rugby (union), football (soccer), concussion

1. Background

Concussions, described as a traumatically induced disturbance of brain function involving complex pathophysiological processes, are a major concern in a number of contact and collision sports. Multiple concussions can be referred to as cumulative mild head injury (CMHI), and are problematic particularly if athletes have competed from a very young age. There is a concern about the sequelae of repeated concussions which has gained prominence in sports psychology [1].

Rugby union and football are examples of designated contact sports where this occurs as a result of collision injuries and in football because of repeated heading of the ball [2]. Rugby union (hereafter referred to as rugby) players (both backs and forwards) are involved in tackling where head to head, head to body or head to ground impact occurs also resulting in concussive injury [3].

Various kinds of head injury occur ranging from severe to mild. Traumatic Brain Injury (TBI) refers to a catastrophic event in which a closed or open head-injury results in serious neural damage which causes permanent cognitive damage [4]. Lack of oxygen to the brain (anoxia) and Cerebrovascular Accidents (CVAs), commonly called 'strokes,' also fall under TBIs.

This chapter focuses on CMHI in the contact sports soccer (hereafter referred to as football) and rugby union (rugby). A description of CMHI will be undertaken however, in order to contextualise this properly TBI and MHI (sometimes called Mild Traumatic Brain Injury—MTBI) will be described. After this a brief review of research, referring to international studies generally and South African studies in particular will be undertaken with specific reference to those involving the author(s).

Nonetheless, international studies on rugby, football and other contact sports are included. It must be noted that this is a complex topic which, cannot be covered comprehensively in a chapter, thus it is a contextual overview of the subject.

1.1 Head injury

Traumatic Brain Injury (TBI) is a catastrophic brain injury. The vast majority of TBIs are closed meaning that the brain is not exposed (the skull is not opened). Closed head injuries (CHIs) are usually called blunt head trauma injuries. This means that the skull can have a fracture but the injury is still closed. Penetrating head injuries (PHIs) are referred to as open head injuries. PHI can include injuries from any source in which the skull and dura are penetrated. The term TBI also encompasses other aetiologies for instance, CVAs (cerebrovascular accidents or strokes) and lack of oxygen to the brain (anoxia) which can be catastrophic [4].

1.2 Frontal lobes of the brain

The frontal lobes of the brain are very vulnerable to damage because of their position (at the front of the head = forehead). Damage to these lobes can be caused by illness (for instance, viral meningitis) or any kind of head injury from a blow to the head caused by a fall, being hit with an object or repeated blows to the head (for instance, in a sport such as boxing). A blow to another part of the head can also cause damage to the frontal lobes of the brain. This happens because the brain is not attached to the inside of the skull and moves around when a head injury is incurred. When the skull hits the back of the head the brain moves and hits the bony protuberances in the skull. This causes bruising (or bleeding) in the brain from slight to catastrophic, depending on the force of the blow to the skull [4, 5]. **Figure 1** is used to illustrate where the frontal lobes of the brain lie illustrating their larger size, which makes them vulnerable to damage from multiple contexts for instance, MVAs (Motor Vehicle Accidents), to illness (Meningitis) and/or sporting injuries (Concussion and CMHIs).

1.3 Open head injury

An open head injury occurs when the skull is penetrated by force which results in a perforated skull [5]. Damage that is incurred is usually in the pathway of the foreign object which often results in the exposure of the intra-dural contents of the brain [6]. Damage may occur because of tangential injuries when something strikes the skull and bone fragments are driven into the brain. These objects may pass through the brain or become embedded in it for instance, bullets causing either/or entrance and exit wounds [5]. There is specific neurological symptomology associated with different types of wounds in this regard [7]. For instance, severe scalp wounds resulting in loss-of-blood may cause low blood pressure (hypotension) and gunshot wounds can cause severe bruises in the brain (contusions) particularly where the enter and leave the skull (countercoup sites). The brain swells and fill with blood and intracranial haematomas can occur [4–6] (**Figure 2**).

1.4 Closed head injury

There are various causes of closed-head injury however, the most common cause is when the skull is injured and the brain suffers acceleration or deceleration and/or both [8]. This can happen in sport for instance, when the skull is hit by something moving quickly such as ball or bat of some kind. This type of accident commonly

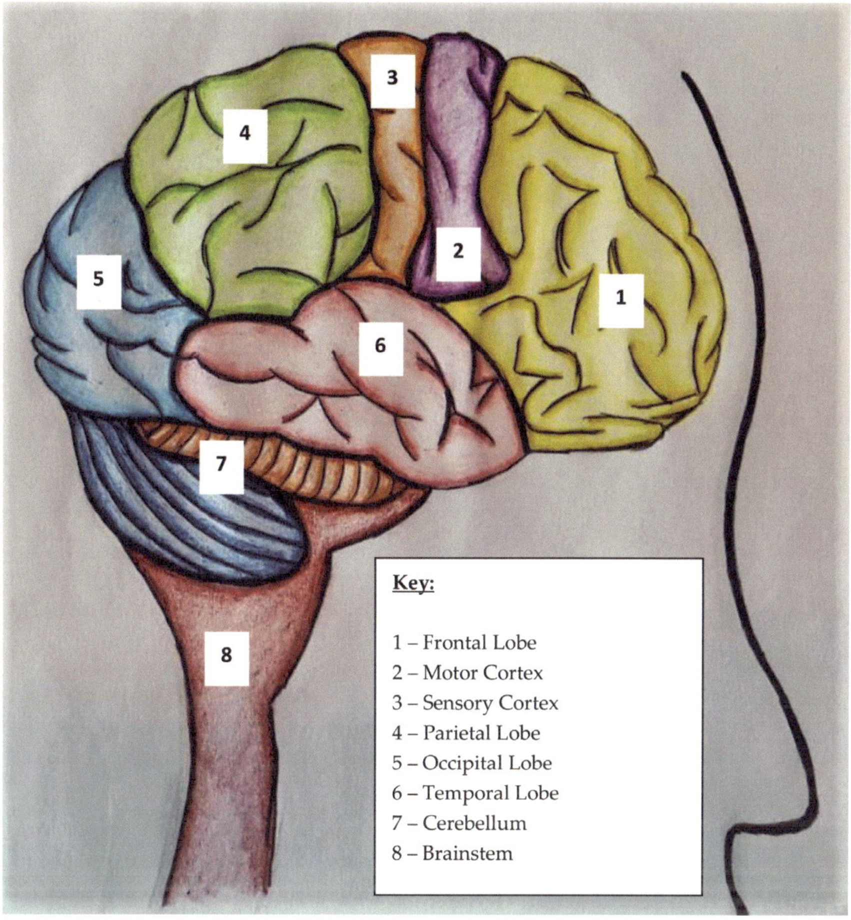

Figure 1.
Lobes of the brain.

occurs in MVAs when a fast moving vehicle stops suddenly which can cause anything from mild to massive brain trauma. However, repeated blows to the head in sport can cause mild brain injury (CMHI) which can be chronic rather than acute and, as a result, the injury effects may not be noticed [9, 10] (**Figure 3**).

1.5 Mild head injury (MHI)

Mild head injury (MHI) and its effects are controversial particularly with regard to definition and classification. For instance, the classification of mild to moderate head injuries is problematic in the research field [11]. MHI refers to an injury in which loss of consciousness (LOC) and/or Post Traumatic Amnesia (PTA) is quite brief and where there is no pathology (or noticeable injury) to the skull [12]. Criterion used to define MHI is underpinned by states of consciousness defined by the Glasgow Coma Scale (GCS) [13]. Problematically, when these are used to define CMHI or MHIs they are unreliable. A classification of MHI in terms of a LOC lasting 30 minutes or less, which is not linked to more neurological symptomology, is often used [14].

A broader definition of MHI includes different grades of injury and: (a) any period of LOC for less than 30 minutes, with GCS of 13–15 following the LOC; (b) any loss of memory for events immediately before or after the accident with

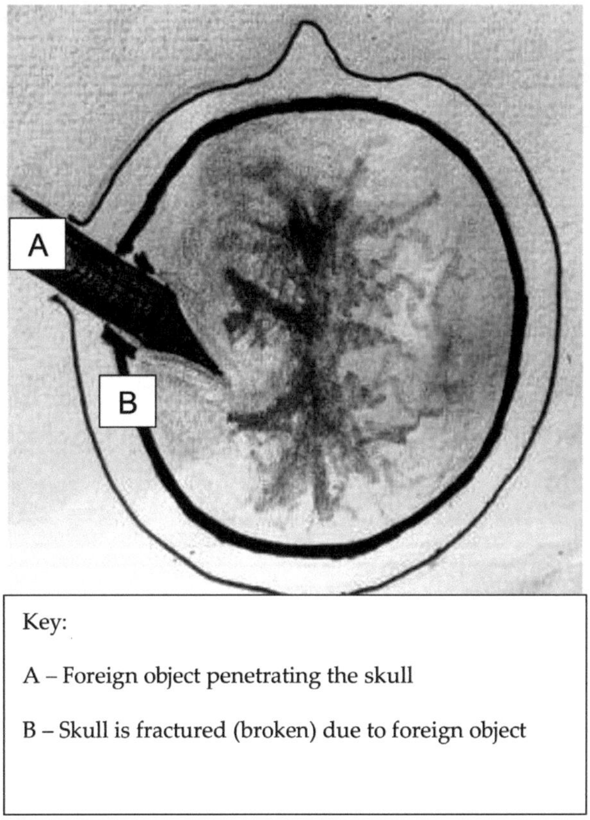

Figure 2.
Schematic diagram of an open head injury.

PTA of less than 24 hours; (c) any alteration in mental state at the time of the accident (for instance, double vision, loss of balance, taste or smell) that may or may not be transient [11].

1.6 Cumulative mild head injury (CMHI)

There is increasing evidence that CMHI can cause more neuropsychological impairment as a result of neural attrition, which can cause athletes problems later in life [15]. Cumulative damage to hippocampal cells can cause cognitive damage [16]. Moreover, CMHI which occurs over months or years is likely to cause neurological and cognitive deficits [17]. The effects of MHI and concussions in the sporting arena are likely cumulative which has significant implications for athletes who play contact sports where concussion and CMHI occur frequently [18, 19]. Research suggests that permanent cognitive deficits are increasing as a result of CMHI [20].

1.7 Concussive injuries (Concussion)

Concussion is any head injury which causes headaches and/or changed levels of consciousness. Fundamentally, an immediate change in neurological functioning because of a blow or injury to the head which results in diffuse axonal injuries (DAI) in the brain structures [20]. This suggests that even short-lived impairment to neural function, after a head injury resulting in a LOC or alteration of consciousness, disturbance of vision and/or equilibrium, is referred to as a concussion. Concerns about the various concussion categories making medical and other research

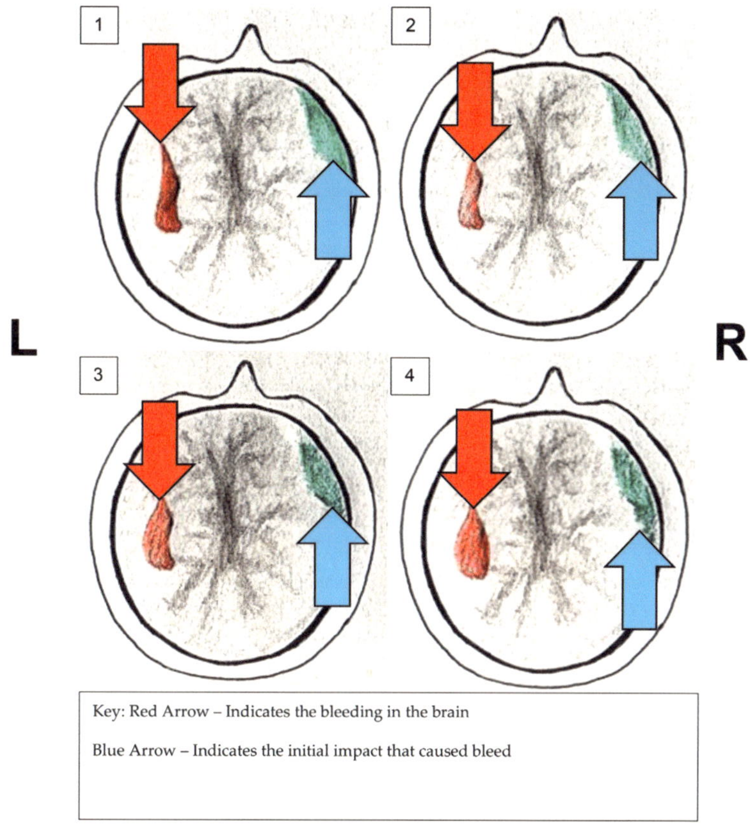

Figure 3.
Schematic representation of a closed head injury.

difficult resulted in guidelines for cerebral concussion [21]. Grade 1 (mild) = transient confusion; no loss of consciousness with symptoms resolving in 15 minutes or less: Grade 2 (moderate) = transient confusion, no loss of consciousness and symptoms lasting longer than 15 minutes and lastly, Grade 3 (severe): any loss of consciousness (brief or prolonged) [22].

The authors in this chapter often use terms like concussion, mild head injury (MHI), mild traumatic brain injury (MBTI) and cumulative mild head injury (CMHI) interchangeably as in the sporting arena to all intent and purpose they often refer to the same thing depending on the sporting code and/or country the injury.

At the first International Conference of Concussion it was stated that concussion was a complex pathophysiological caused by biochemical forces impacting on the brain [23]. The definition included the following concussion: (1) may be caused by a blow to the head face, neck, or elsewhere with force that is transferred to the brain; (2) characteristically causes the speedy onset of brief impairment of neurological functions that resolve spontaneously; (3) results in neuropathological changes however, acute clinical symptomology reflects functional disturbances as opposed to structural injury; (4) is a set of clinical syndromes that sometimes (but not always) involves a LOC. Symptomology is resolved following a specific sequence and (5) it is characteristically associated with fundamentally normal structural neuroimaging. A later addition to this was that in some cases post-concussive symptoms can be protracted and persistent [19]. It is used to refer to a closed, MHI such as those incurred by athletes who play contact sports. It falls within the ambit of MHI and CMHI and can be difficult to detect as symptoms can last from a few seconds to minutes [5]. In this chapter this type of head injury denotes any impact to the head which often go un-reported (**Figure 4**).

1.8 Occurrence of mild head injury (MHI)

Reliable statistics about the occurrence (prevalence) of MHIs that are closed are quite difficult to ascertain. This is as a result of different names for instance, mild, minor, moderate, and minimal being applied to this type of head injury.

The incidence of MHI is difficult to determine because the majority of country health surveys only look at patients who have been hospitalised. This means that patients who have suffered a MHI or CMHI are not included in survey data. The International Classification of Diseases (ICD 10, 2010) has specific terms of reference for instance, for maxillofacial injuries and scalp lacerations but do not specify CMHI or MHI. Individuals admitted to hospitals who have multiple injuries are usually classified in terms of their most severe injuries (thus an MHI goes unreported [24]).

In South Africa there are few statistics on MHI however, an average of 316 per 100,000 incidents of brain injuries per year was reported in the early nineties [25]. It is estimated for instance, that up to 89,000 brain injuries (mostly TBIs) are seen per year in the country [26]. Moreover, rugby has the highest incidence of concussion amongst contact sport with up to 50% of athletes suffering from a concussion in their playing careers [11].

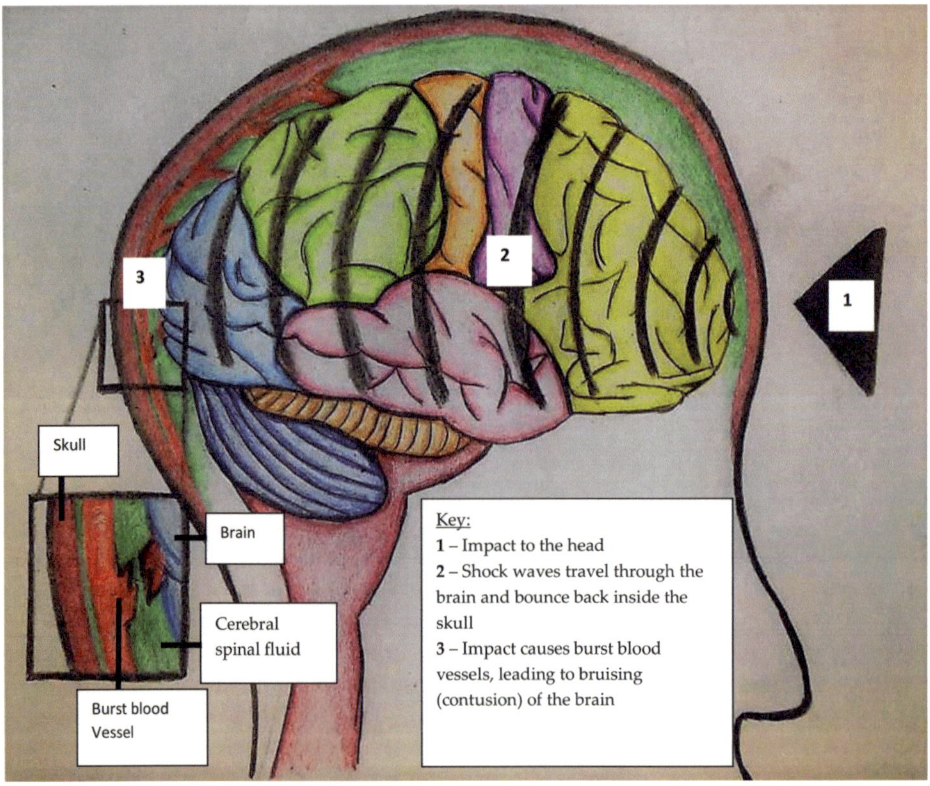

Figure 4.
Schematic representation of how a concussion occurs.

1.9 The mechanics of mild head injury (MHI)

Mild head injury (MHI) involves primary and secondary brain injury. Primary injury occurs on impact and secondary injury occurs after the impact. Secondary brain injury can stem from complications arising out of a primary brain injury. The time-span in which secondary damage can be from seconds, minutes to hours and/or days after the first injury [27].

1.10 Primary brain injury

The contact force is the major origin of brain damage in so-called still injuries where an immobile victim receives a blow to the head. The knock to the head results in movement of the head and neck on impact and causes angular acceleration, a combination of translational and rotational acceleration [5]. Cerebral bruises or contusions are made up of focal damage to the brain tissue which can result in a tear or laceration as a result of head trauma. The coup is an injury that results from a direct blow to the head and appears below the site of impact. A countercoup is when the brain sustains contusion(s) in an area opposite the blow which occurs mostly in the frontal and temporal lobes [5].

The major theories which explain countercoup injuries are: (1) vibration or Echo theory which states that the traumatic impact sets up vibrations which are reflected in damage to the opposite pole of the brain; (2) Transmitted Force Theory which suggests that traumatic impact results in a transmission of applied force through brain tissue which causes the contralateral structures of the brain to be pushed against the inside of the skull; (3) Brain Displacement Theory which posits that countercoup injuries are a result of avulsion of the cerebral cortex from the overlying meninges; (4) Pressure Gradient Theory suggests that when there is a sudden fall in intracranial pressure, opposite to the point of impact, blood vessels rupture; and (5) Rotational Theory posits that after a blow to the skull the brain is set in a centrifugal motion in line with the direction of the original force or impact. The brain is then thrust against the bony protuberances on the interior of the skull [4].

1.11 Secondary brain injury

Secondary brain injury occurs at different lengths of time after head trauma. It is important to recognise that Mild Traumatic Brain Injury (MTBI) is a dynamic process as the symptomology and pathology evolves hourly and sometimes days after an injury occurs [28]. In fact, much of the brain damage which eventually ensues is as a result of the secondary injury [1]. Hypoxia or low oxygen to the brain and/or insufficient blood supply (ischemia) are the mechanisms through which it suffers an insult [29]. Haematoma, oedema (swelling) in the white matter of the brain next to focal mass lesions, intracranial haemorrhage, diffuse brain swelling, ischaemic brain damage, raised intracranial pressure, brain shift and herniation are other conditions which cause secondary brain injury [28]. Furthermore, although far less common, the risk of Second Impact Syndrome (SIS), a very serious and even fatal brain injury may occur even after a relatively mild impact, which can be significant in young rugby players. SIS occurs when an athlete suffers a concussion and before the first injury has recovered suffers another injury to the head. In SIS it is possible for rapid deterioration and even death. This happens because the brain has not recovered from the first injury and the second injury results in rapid swelling and pressure within the skull. This intracranial pressure, if uncontrolled, can lead to death [30].

1.12 The pathophysiology of mild head injury (MHI) and CMHI

1.12.1 Diffuse Axonal Injury (DAI)

Diffuse Axonal Injury (DAI) is caused through acceleration-deceleration trauma when the brain twists or rotates inside the skull (rotational acceleration). Focally diffuse axonal strain and tensile stress results in one of the most compromising types of injury in brain trauma [31]. Fundamentally, after a serious head injury it is probably the major cause of unconsciousness and persistent vegetative states. It was first described in the late 1950s after post-mortems conducted on individuals who had died as a result of severe head trauma [32]. This kind of injury has a serious impact on the executive functioning of the brain and alters for instance, the speed of information processing, working memory and attention span [4]. It is postulated that DAI is involved in persistent post-concussive symptomology and attentional deficits following MTBI [33] (**Figure** 5).

1.13 Post-concussive syndrome (PCS)

Minor impacts to the head cause a pattern of self-reported symptomology referred to as post-concussive syndrome (PCS). These symptoms can persist long after the original injury, and can be both acute and/or chronic. They are categorised into three main symptom areas: cognitive, physical and psychological [34]. Although symptoms generally resolve within a period of a week to 3 months there can be chronic symptomology which occurs from months to years after the initial trauma [5]. These reactions to MHI are facilitated by various issues and are based on an interaction between organic and psychological factors basically, they begin at an organic level and sometimes persist and are experienced at a psychological level. Somatic symptomology includes dizziness, tiredness and headaches whereas psychological symptomology is related to: poor concentration and memory; irritability, emotional lability and depression and anxiety [4].

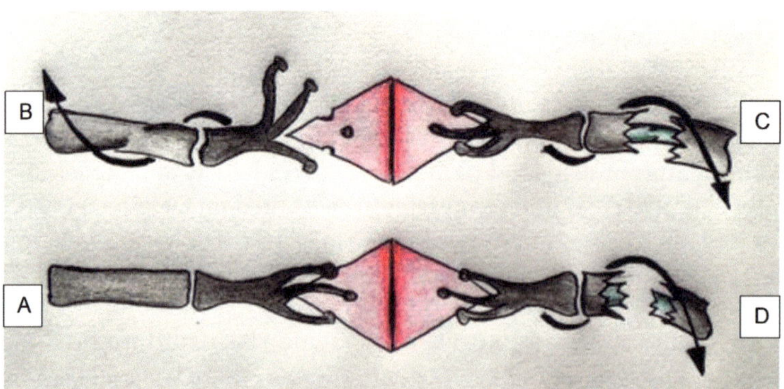

Key:

A – Normal Axon with connection

B – Twisted Axon (pulled away at the synapse end)

C – Torn Axon

D – Broken Axon

Figure 5.
Schematic representation of a diffuse axonal injury.

In the sporting arena there are various physical and neurological symptoms experienced by athletes for instance, headaches and dizziness, impaired concentration and memory plus poor problem solving ability. This type of symptomology may be based on personality characteristics in athletes or be related to malingering and/or the possibility of financial gain [5].

1.13.1 Post-concussive syndrome (PCS) diagnostic criteria

The two most commonly cited systems for defining and diagnosing PCS are the 10th edition of the International Classification of Disease [35] and the Diagnostic and Statistical Manual of Mental Disorders—DSM-5 [36]. In this chapter we present the ICD-10 (2010) diagnostic criteria as it is more universally applied and many individuals do not meet the DSM-5 criteria pertaining to cognitive deficits and clinically significant criteria (which can also be problematic in terms of finding incidence and prevalence of PCS): (a) history of head trauma with loss of consciousness precedes symptoms onset by maximum of 4 weeks and (b) symptoms in three or more of the following categories:

- Headache, dizziness, malaise, fatigue, noise tolerance;
- Irritability, depression, anxiety, emotional lability;
- Subjective concentration, memory, or intellectual difficulties without neuropsychological evidence of marked improvement impairment;
- Insomnia;
- Reduced alcohol tolerance;
- Preoccupation with above symptoms and fear of brain damage with hypochondriacal concerns and adoption of sick role.

The grading of concussions is also important in this regard see **Table 1** [22].

1.13.2 Recovery and symptomology related to post-concussive syndrome (PCS)

Diagnosis of PCS is based on the subjective symptomology reported by individuals as is recovery (based on symptom resolution) [5]. Adults' cognitive deficits and symptoms in terms of PCS are commonly found in the acute stage and resolve within 3–12 months [37]. The duration of amnesia related to any LOC is also very important [4] (**Table 2**).

Grade of Concussion	Severity of Concussion	Symptoms
Grade 1	Mild	Temporary Confusion No Loss of Consciousness (LOC) Symptoms resolve in less than 15 minutes
Grade 2	Moderate	Temporary Confusion No LOC Symptoms last longer than 15 minutes
Grade 3	Severe	Any LOC (transitory or protracted)

Table 1.
Concussion grading.

Time of Amnesia	Severity
Less than 5 minutes	Very Mild
Five (5) to sixty (60) minutes	Mild
One (1) to twenty-four (24) hours	Moderate
One (1) to seven (7) days	Severe
One (1) to four (4) weeks	Very Severe

Table 2.
Post traumatic amnesia.

MHI symptomology are often non-specific and may be the same as those reported after for instance, orthopaedic injuries. The most frequently reported symptoms are headaches, blurred vision, dizziness, subjective memory problems and sleep disturbance [35] (**Table 3**).

Return to play protocols for professional athletes in football and rugby are the norm and well-defined (see **Tables 4** and **5**) but this is not the case in the amateur spheres of the game where injuries may be more severe because of the poorer skill levels of the athletes [38].

1.14 Neuropsychological sequelae of mild head injuries (MHIs)

Individuals who sustain MTBI often report symptomology comparative with PCS. It has been reported that 10–20% of MTBI patients report PCS that go beyond a recovery period of 6–12 months [39]. Severe tiredness (up to 50% of individuals who report PCS) is often reported which impacts on an individual's cognitive ability and can cause day-to-day problems in living relating to work, exercise and sports participation as well as social interactions. Psychological symptomology for instance, depression is also associated with MHIs as well as anxiety and irritability [40]. Children who experience MHI are more likely to experience impulse control problems and, as a result, have poorer planning ability. They are at a higher risk of difficulty with high-level cognitive functions [41]. As many children and adolescents play rugby and football this is a problematic finding.

1.14.1 Changes to the neurochemical make-up of the brain after a head injury

Neurochemical change as a result of head injury is facilitated by damaged brain cells and occurs within an hour and up to 10 days post-injury [18]. This creates a metabolic dysfunction which means there is an imbalance between the demand of

	Criteria
1.	History of Head trauma with loss of consciousness precedes symptoms onset by maximum of four weeks
2.	Symptoms in three or more of the following symptom categories: • Headache, dizziness, malaise, fatigue, noise tolerance. • Irritability, depression, anxiety, emotional lability. • Subjective concentration, memory, or intellectual difficulties without neuropsychological evidence of marked improvement impairment. • Insomnia. • Reduced alcohol tolerance. • Preoccupation with above symptoms and fear of brain damage with hypochondriacal concerns and adaption of sick role.

Table 3.
ICD10 post concussive criteria.

<table>
<tr><th colspan="2">When a player shows any symptoms or signs of concussion.</th><th>The following shall be applied for Acute Injury:</th></tr>
<tr><td colspan="2">1.</td><td>The player should not be allowed to return to play in the current game or practice.</td></tr>
<tr><td colspan="2">2.</td><td>The player should be left alone, and regular monitoring for deterioration is essential over the initial few hours after injury.</td></tr>
<tr><td colspan="2">3.</td><td>The player should be medically evaluated after the injury.</td></tr>
<tr><td colspan="2">4.</td><td>Return to play must follow a medically supervised stepwise process.</td></tr>
<tr><td colspan="2">NB: A player should never return to play while symptomatic</td><td>"When in doubt, sit them out"</td></tr>
<tr><th>Level</th><th>Return to play protocols
Activity undertaken</th><th>Time Post-Concussion
(Approx. guidelines)</th></tr>
<tr><td>1.</td><td>No Activity, complete rest, once symptom free and cognitive recovery is demonstrated, proceed to level 2.</td><td>2 – 3 Days</td></tr>
<tr><td>2.</td><td>Light aerobic exercise, such as walking or stationary cycling.</td><td>4 – 10 Days</td></tr>
<tr><td>3.</td><td>Sport specific training, such as running, drills, ball handling skills.</td><td>11 – 15 Days</td></tr>
<tr><td>4.</td><td>Non-contact training drills</td><td>16 – 20 Days</td></tr>
<tr><td>5.</td><td>Full Contact training after medical clearance</td><td>21 Days</td></tr>
<tr><td>6.</td><td>Game play</td><td>21+ Days</td></tr>
</table>

Table 4.
Management of concussion and return to play protocols.

Number of Stages	Rehabilitation Stage	Functional exercise at each stage of rehabilitation	Objective of each stage of Protocol
1.	No activity	Complete physical and cognitive rest	Recovery
2.	Light aerobic activity	Walking, swimming or stationary cycling keeping intensity <70% of maximum. No resistance training	Increase Heart Rate
3.	Sport-specific exercise	Running drills in soccer No head impact exercises	Add movement
4.	Non-contact training drills	Progression to more complex training e.g. passing drills in football. May start progressive resistance training	Exercise, co-ordination and cognitive load
5.	Full contact practice	Following medical clearance participate in normal training	Restore confidence and assessment of functional skills by coaching staff
6.	Return to play	Normal game play	

Table 5.
Graduated return to play protocol.

the brain for energy (to heal itself) and for it to work at its usual capacity. This may be one of the reasons for SIS. The protein S-100 has been found at higher than normal levels for around a year after MHIs which impairs neurological functioning in the brain [42].

1.14.2 Imbalances in hormones after a head injury

Damage to the hypothalamus and/or the pituitary gland can cause hormonal problems as these glands regulate hormones in the body [4]. Changes in sexual function, depression, headaches and tiredness may occur. As these are also linked to concussive injury, hormonal damage can be overlooked. In one study after severe

TBIs abnormal hormone levels were found in 60% of patients [43]. This could occur in some cases of MHI and CMHI (**Figure 6**).

1.15 Neuropsychological recovery following mild and cumulative mild head injuries (CMHI)

Some pundits suggest that acute sequelae resolution of any MHI neuropsychological deficits takes from 4 to 5 weeks post the initial head trauma but that there still might be problems with psychosocial capabilities. These can be mild cognitive insufficiencies related to slower information processing and slower visuomotor speed. Deficits pertaining to tiredness, dizziness and headaches often reduce after a period of 2 months post-injury but some patients still report PCS 3 months post-injury. These symptoms are often mild and may go unnoticed at medical follow-ups [34]. Return to play protocols are thus very important [38].

1.16 Neuropsychological assessment of deficits related to CMHI

In the mid-1980s medical and allied health professionals started neuropsychological testing [22] because head injuries in professional sports (especially contact sports) were noted as potentially keeping the athlete of the field of play (and sport requires its sporting heroes in order to make money). A number of high profile professional athletes who played American Football incurred head injuries and did

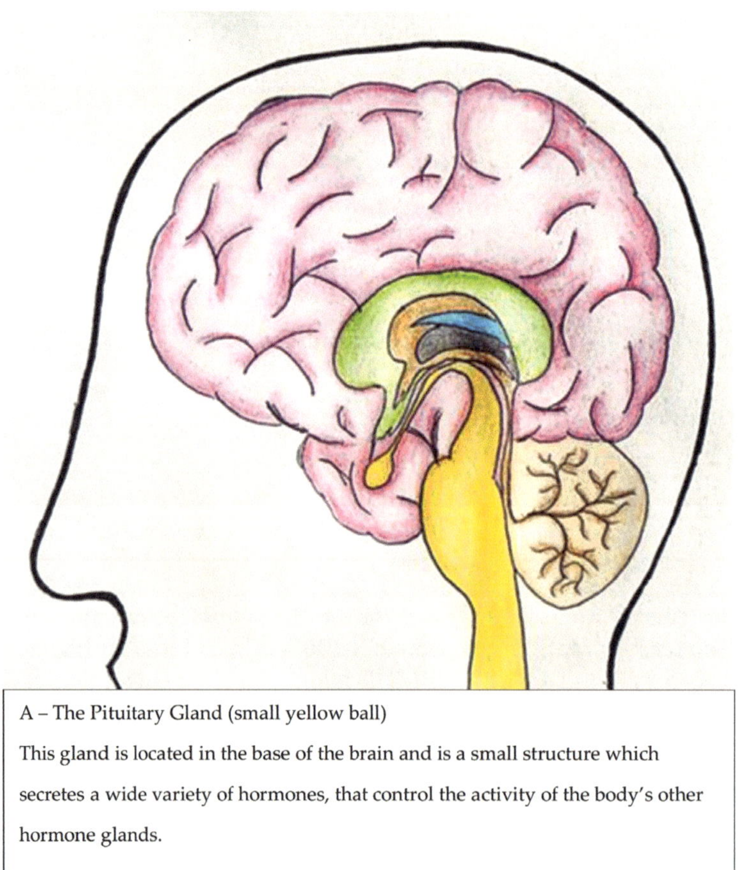

Figure 6.
The pituitary gland.

not recover timeously, costing their franchises much money. As a result baseline neuropsychological testing was used by several major American Football franchises. The National Hockey League (NHL) in the United States of America (USA) authorised this type of testing for comparable reasons. Baseline neuropsychological testing has, since then, become the norm in some countries in collegiate and professional sport and has allowed post injury evaluation of subtle cognitive functions linked to CMHIS. In turn, this data has supported intervention (and treatment) protocols for various professional sporting codes [4].

This suggests that the assessment of cognitive functions is critical in terms of amateur and professional sport particularly in contact sports, and should include baseline cognitive and postural stability testing for athletes in high-risk contact sports [44, 45].

Different types of attention can be assessed using various neuropsychological tests for instance, arousal and alertness can be evaluated using an electroencephalography spectral analysis because the hippocampal theta rhythm is linked to heightened attention [5]. Selective attention can be assessed by using different neuropsychological measures such as hemi-spatial inattention using Line Bisection, Letter cancellation, and the drawing of symmetrical figures. Focused attention can be assessed using the Stroop Color and Word Test. Fundamentally, focused attention is usually evaluated in the visual and auditory areas by utilising dichotic listening tasks. In this type of test an individual listens to various kinds of auditory stimuli and is asked to make specific choices. Other tests of focused attention are the Letter Cancellation Task, the Trail Making Tests and Reaction Time with Distraction tests. Divided attention deficits are usually seen by lower speeds in performance tasks and assessed using for instance, the Paced Auditory Serial Addition Test where the degree of deficit compares positively with the severity of injury. Individuals suffering mild concussion have been found to be up to three times slower than control group individuals with no concussive injury. Athletes who experienced severe concussion were found to be up to five times slower than control group members with no concussive injury. Sustained attention deficits can be seen as time-on-task deficits. In other words, an individual takes longer than the norm to complete a task. Other neuropsychological tests for sustained attention are for instance, the Letter cancellation test, Vigilance tests and Perceptual Speed tests [4, 5].

Computerised cognitive tests (CCTS) are available that evaluate changes in cognition [46]. For instance, the Post-Concussion Assessment and Cognitive Test (ImPACT). These can be more accurate than pen-paper tests but qualitative data from interviewing patients must also be used to give a complete report on any head injured athlete.

1.17 Reaction time related to head injuries

Reaction time (RT) is the period in milliseconds from when a test stimulus is presented to the time the individual reacts. In simple RT testing (using a computerised programme) there is only one stimulus and one response which measures psychomotor skills [46]. In choice RT testing the testee gives a response when presented with a stimulus on the computer screen [4]. Computerised assessment is more accurate than older pen-paper tests and, because of high overall use of smart phones and computers, all populations are able to complete these tests [45]. The two critical measurements taken during this type of assessment are reaction time (RT) and movement time (MT). RT, according to some pundits, reflects decision time which is defined as the length of time for stimulus evaluation and response programming. Conversely, movement time (MT), is the measure of the time it takes to complete a response. RT is reflective of cognitive processes while

MT is linked to the motor component of the RT. RT can be defined as the sum of RT and MT which equals Total Reaction Time. Good RT is needed by athletes in order to perform well in any given sporting code and a head injury, which results in poorer RT, is a challenge (caused by for instance, CMHI, MHI). Factors that influence good RT are high stimulation, tiredness, alcohol consumption and any type of brain injury [45].

1.18 Use of neuroimaging techniques in diagnosing MHI deficits

Traditional neuroimaging devices for instance, Magnetic Resonance Imaging (MRI) and Computerised Tomography (CT) scans are not appropriate for MHI and CMHI as they do not pick up the pathophysiological processes in this type of head injury [18]. However, newer structural MRIs which include gradient echo perfusion and diffusion imaging are more sensitive to structural abnormalities so may be more useful [19]. Traditional neuropsychological assessments (pen and paper and computerised tests) have proven their usefulness in diagnosing MHI deficits and are very sensitive to diffuse axonal damage thus are used successfully in the sporting environment.

1.19 Cross-cultural neurological assessment

The culture and ethnicity of an athlete must be looked at carefully when interpreting data from any kind of neuropsychological/neurological assessments. Many of these tests have not been standardised on people from non-westernised Caucasian backgrounds which could prove problematic. Construct equivalence for the assessment of individuals who are not from the culture that a test has been standardised and validated on usually does not exist. The assessment of an athlete's responses on a neurological/neuropsychological evaluation must take into account their socio-cultural context and experiences [4, 5]. If these are overlooked there may be a culturally inappropriate analysis which can result in false positive or false negative results.

1.20 Examples of research on CMHI in the contact sports rugby union, rugby 7s and football

Cumulative mild head injury (CMHI) research, to a large extent, has been conducted on rugby union players. Players are fit, the forwards are heavy (up to 140 kg) and it is described as a very physical sport [4]. Although the sport originated in, and was initially played, in Europe it is a very popular sport in the southern hemisphere (for instance in Australia (AUS), South Africa (SA) and New Zealand (NZ)). It is becoming increasingly popular in Japan and the USA which has prompted more research in the field.

In 2000 an investigation looked at the cumulative effects of concussion and CMHI on professional rugby players. A group of 26 professional rugby players and a control group of non-contact sports (professional cricketers) athletes was used. In the rugby group forward and backline players were compared over a neuropsychological test-battery. Results indicated that rugby players, particularly the forwards, had deficits in verbal, working and visual memory as well as visuoperceptual tracking skills as compared to the cricket playing controls. It was also found that within the rugby group mean score test comparisons indicated that the forwards displayed greater cognitive deficits than the backline players [47]. Conversely, research into intellectual deficits incurred by CMHI in high school rugby players, revealed no significant association between the actual reported MHIs and intellectual or cognitive dysfunction [48].

In 2001 an investigation into CMHI amongst schoolboy rugby players and a hockey playing control group revealed more variability, on a battery of neuropsychological tests, amongst the forward rugby playing group (as compared to the backline rugby players) as well as the hockey playing group. Working memory and visuospatial processing skills were more impaired in the rugby forwards than the backline and hockey players and the entire rugby playing sample showed more of these deficits than the hockey playing control group [49].

Enduring PCS amongst school boys and adult players (at the national level) was looked at using visuomotor processing speed tests. Results suggested that the rugby playing group had less capability on various tests post-season. It was postulated that this was probably due to unreported concussions and/or the cumulative effect of mild head injuries. It was also reported that the rugby forwards (who engage in more scrummaging and heavy tackling) showed more cognitive deficits than the rugby backline players [50].

In 2010 an investigation, using a neuropsychological test battery, was carried out into the effects of three or more concussive injuries in adult male rugby players. It was found that rugby players who had suffered multiple concussive injuries performed lower on the test-battery than those who had no previous history of concussion. The results suggested that rugby players who had incurred three or more concussions were likely to suffer cognitive dysfunction [3].

On the other hand, an investigation into CMHI using computerised testing, on a sample of high school rugby players, did not support research which indicates that concussive injury and/or CMHI results in cognitive deficits. The major body of research in SA indicates that CMHI results in some cognitive deficits particularly in rugby forwards. In this research neither rugby forwards or backs showed cognitive dysfunction post-season relative to the hockey controls. It was anticipated that, as the computerised test was very sensitive to diffuse brain injury, some cognitive dysfunction would be found. The research concluded that perhaps MHIs in this group (adolescent boys) does not have a cumulative effect as previously postulated. It was also suggested that factors such as education and age may mitigate against CMHI [9] however, as this was a small sample results were considered provisional [51].

Conversely, a small 2017 study looking at CMHI in college rugby union players found that there was significant variability on mean scores between rugby frontline and backline players on verbal memory, concept formation, cognitive flexibility, working memory and visual-motor processing speed on a pen-paper neuropsychological test battery. In this research it was postulated that poor scores on PCS might also indicate depression in the rugby playing group as insomnia and anger were frequently reported [52].

An Australian study found that in a sample of 104 amateur rugby sevens players (males and females) in one season thirty-one injuries occurred. These were mostly caused by contact at speed and tackling. In the investigation it was noted that head, neck and shoulder injuries made up 50% of all injuries however, CMHI was not investigated. It was reported that athletes that were slower and less agile were at more risk of injury as were female 7s players. The study concluded that there are limited studies on risks factors associated with rugby sevens player and that more pre and post season assessment was required [53].

A study on school level rugby union players in Australia looked at 332 injuries in different age ranges over a season (10–18 years). It was found that the incidence of supposed concussion injuries was 4.3/1000 players and that the most usual way of incurring this injury was tacking. Risk factors were that the game itself is a physically challenging contact sport where many tackles are made at high speed. Over a third of injuries in this sample were to the head and face and overall there were 61 reported concussion. As this was a high incidence it was recommend that prevention programmes need to be put in place [54].

A recent study in Ireland looking at recurrent injuries in teenage rugby in 15–18 year olds (15–18 years) found that recurrent injuries numbered 426. Eighty-one concussions were reported of these, 5% were recurrent (in the season under investigation). Although these were the lowest number of recurrent injuries it was noted that any concussive injury that occurs on multiple occasions could be potentially disastrous [55]. In this regard the evaluation and management of concussive injury in young contact sports players is very important because they may have a long-term effect on the athletes to heal [56, 57] for instance, the development of chronic traumatic encephalopathy [55].

There has been very little research into CMHI in football (soccer) players in South Africa. Originally the sport was a non-contact sport but the contemporary game is a designated contact sport [4]. It has been reported that concussive injuries in football are often not reported (players do not wish to leave the field as they do not want to be 'benched' for 6 weeks or until recovery) and, as a result, are under-diagnosed [4]. Athletes involved in football may incur head-to-head, head-to-ground (or post) and head-to-ball injuries thus there is the likelihood of CMHI. Although head-to-ball injuries may seem unlikely a ball kicked at half-speed travels between 22 and 83 km an hour and can hit the skull with a force of 116 km an hour [59]. A full powered kick could hit the head at around 200 km an hour. As there are about five possibilities a match for any team member to head the ball [60], there is the possibility of CMHI. As early as 1989 research concluded that 12 of 37 football players in a study had slightly abnormal or abnormal EEG (Electroencephalograph) results compared to only 4 of 37 controls who had never played football [58].

In 1989 a study in Norway found that football players self-reported symptoms of irritability, inability to sleep, poor working memory, dizziness, neck pain and headaches after they had repeatedly headed the ball [58]. This supported another 1993 study using male and female Olympic football players. In this research 55% of female and 54% of male football players in the sample reported concussive symptomology after repeated headings of the ball [59]. These investigations underpin earlier findings in 1983 where it was reported that out of every 10 football players 2 had abnormal EEGs when they had trained for 15 minutes in heading the ball [60]. There is concern that youngsters who play football from an early age, and repeatedly head the ball (or are involved in collisions), can have cognitive deficits in later life, possibly as a result of CMHI and concussive injury in the game [4, 61].

Conversely, a study in 2000 reported no acute cognitive deficits in a sample of male and female football players and any significant differences were reported as due to practice effects [62]. However, a 2001 study did find cognitive dysfunction relating to memory and planning abilities in amateur football players in an American college sample [18]. On the other hand, it was reported that concussion from head to ground injuries and collisions were more likely to cause this type of brain injury than repeated heading of the ball [63].

A 2016 study in South Africa looking at sample football players and a control group of non-contact sport athletes (volleyball) using a computerised assessment package (measuring reaction time) and looking at PCS found the following: pre-season volleyball players actually had a better (or faster) reaction time than the football players (not significant). Post-season on a test of simple reaction time there were no significant differences. Both groups reaction times improved in relation to their pre-season results. This may suggest that playing these sports and engaging in reaction time training actually improves and develops athletes reaction times. As this was computerised testing any diffuse brain damage should have been seen in the results, this was not the case as no significant deficits in football players were found. Conversely, on PCS over a quarter of the football players and only 6% of the control group experienced symptoms such as headaches, attention problems, memory problems, irritation, nervousness and anxiety. This may suggest that athletes involved in football do sustain some CMHI and/or concussive injury which is not reflected in their reaction time scores. This was a small sample of 15 footballers and 15 volleyball controls thus results are provisional [64].

A 2016 study looking at concussion in elite male football players found that this type of injury was a risk factor for incurring another such injury within a year of the first injury. Interestingly, the athletes who had a previous concussive injury also had more other injuries than the non-concussed football players in the study. It was suggested that this may be caused by the type of behaviour these athletes engage in (on the field of play) and due to their inherent personality characteristics [65].

The aforementioned literature indicates why there is a debate in football as to whether young players should be allowed to head the ball [66] particularly if tiredness has an impact on performance [67].

1.21 Recent literature concussive injuries in other sporting codes

This section will present several studies related to head injuries in other sporting codes so that the reader is made aware of the extent of these injuries in the sporting arena today.

Combat sports such as wrestling, mixed martial arts, taekwondo incur many injuries which are mostly soft-tissue and contusion injuries, however, a meta-review found that 15% of injuries in these sports are concussive in nature (90% classified as mild to moderate). Risk factors include age, weight category, experience, training and gender, females more likely to incur this type of injury [68].

Cricket players, although the sport is usually designated a non-contact sport, can also receive craniofacial and head injuries if they are hit by a cricket ball (usually when batting). Although using a helmet helped with neck and head injuries it is possible for possible head injuries to occur [69]. Furthermore, another review which looked at craniofacial injuries between 1870 and 2015 found a relatively small number (36). However, 5 resulted in a fatal injury and 9 resulted in the cricketer no longer being able to play the game. In this study it was also reported that in some instance concussion was difficult to diagnosed. It was concluded that all cricket clubs should have medical professionals available and that concussive injuries needed early identification and appropriate management [70].

Boxers generally suffer more repetitive chronic traumatic brain injury (CTBI) which is not mild or moderate in nature. However, all repetitive injuries to the brain are cumulative in nature and, in the case of boxing, where many blows to the head are received there is the possibility of SIS. As a result since the early twentieth century boxing careers were, on average, 19 years in length but are now around 5 years long. There are still deaths in the sport however, recent research suggest that CBTI caused by repetitive blows to the head will become fever because of medical interventions such as neuroimaging and the early discovery of these injuries [71].

American football is another sport where there are many concussive injuries as it is a contact sport that is considered both violent and dangerous. In a review of head injuries in the game it was revealed that athletes, who have many concussions are, as they age, at risk of non-resolving cognitive deficits, dementia and depression. Retirement age is not prescribed in the sport however, it was suggested that risk

Risk factors for MHI (CMHI & MTBI)	Impact and/or outcomes
Age	• Young contact sport players as brain development not complete; • Older players of contact sports because of: ➢ Likelihood of repeated MHI; ➢ Less agile and slower reaction times than younger contact sports players.
Gender	• Studies suggest that female contact sport players are more at risk of MHI and concussive injury.
Duration of concussion	• Mild • Moderate • Severe (see table 1)
Duration of Post-Traumatic Amnesia (PTA)	• Very mild • Mild • Moderate • Severe • Very severe (see table 2)
General conditioning of the athlete	• If athlete not fit and overweight high risk factor; • If athlete fit but moving a fast speed and making contact with/or tackling other physically fit players; • Position played within the contact sport for instance, rugby forwards because of tackling and scrummaging may be more at risk than rugby backline players.
Un-reported illness	• Players who have had influenza or other illnesses and who have taken medication are often allowed to play during important games (particularly in the amateur arena). This is a risk factor for injury and MHI.
Overuse of alcohol and/or substances	• These (even over the counter or prescribed substances) put athletes at risk; • In both professional, but particularly amateur, contact sporting codes much alcohol is consumed which is also a risk factor.
Poor skills	• Amateur and young players do not have a full skill-set thus may be more prone to MHI; • Players with poor skill sets may be inclined to be more reckless in their sport of choice facilitating MHI.
Poor or inappropriate training	• Related to the abovementioned bullet – lack of proper or incorrect training techniques in the sport of choice leads to vulnerability to MHI.
Poor concussion management	• Poor concussion management protocols are a high risk factor for repeated injuries and SIS (see table 4).
Poor return to play protocol	• Return to play protocols must be in place and strictly adhered to otherwise the athlete is at risk of CMHI and SIS (see table 5).
The 'blind eye' syndrome	• Coaches and management turning a 'blind eye' to concussive injuries and either allowing or making athletes return to their sport too quickly.
Athlete under-reporting of concussive injury	• Pressure from team management, coaches and possible loss of earnings or losing place in the team facilitates under-reporting of these injuries by athletes.
Non- availability of medical staff	• Professional games are required to have medics however; these are not always available during practices; • In contact sports at amateur level there are often either no trained medical professionals or poor trained allied health professionals; • The abovementioned is the same for school contact sports and during practices there are usually no health professionals present.
No pre and post season testing cognitive (or reaction time) tessting	• In professional sport this is usually carried out on all players (though not always); • In amateur and school sports pre and post season testing for MHI is not usually undertaken. There are many head-impact measurement devices available which may be too expensive for all stakeholders however, pen-paper testing is available.
Unsuitable protective clothing/gear	• Protective clothing of any kind (including helmets) is often not the correct size or incorrectly worn, which is a risk factor; • Second hand protective clothing/gear should not be used as it has lost much of its efficacy; • Many sporting codes do not have rules that protective clothing/gear is worn by a) all players or b) by amateur or young players (for instance, skull caps in rugby and helmets when batting in cricket).
Family history of specific illnesses	• Players of contact sport who have familial histories of: ➢ Depression; ➢ Senile Dementia ➢ And other degenerative diseases, are
	are likely more at risk of early onset of the last two bullets and, at any stage during their sport career, of becoming depressed.

Table 6.
Risk factors in contact sports for cumulative mild head injury (CMI) and concussive injury.

factors for neurocognitive impairment should be taken into account for instance, age, number of concussive injuries, length of time taken to recover and any non-resolving functional deficits [72].

Ice-hockey players are also at risk of concussive head injuries. It was found that young and older players are more at risk due to possible lack of skills and in the latter case tiredness causing them to be more careless in their playing style. Overall, it was concluded that this type of MTBI is serious in nature and more research needs undertaken in this sporting code [73].

There are many risk factors for CMHI and concussive injury in rugby union, rugby 7s, football and other sporting codes. A summary of these is provided in **Table 6**. **Table 6** is not exhaustive but based on the authors reading of the literature.

2. Conclusion

Recently in South Africa (as well as internationally) there has been much interest in research into the neuropsychological sequelae following concussive injuries [1, 50, 51, 61, 63–67]. This type of research is vital in contributing to the field of sports psychology and sports medicine in terms of understanding the clinical features and assessment techniques, clinical management, rehabilitation, education of athletes and their health care providers, return-to play guidelines and long-term outcomes of concussive injuries. Although it is widely believed that athletes are fit to return to play when observed symptoms resolve, researchers continue to investigate the prolonged effects of concussion and repeated concussion on cognitive difficulties, emotional disturbances and behavioural issues.

Acknowledgements

Thanks to Dr. Patricia Maite, Mr. Christopher Nel and Ms. Mokgadi Rapetsoa for their research in the field and Ms. Katy Nel for her original drawings.

Thank you to the University of Limpopo Research Office specifically Director Mabila and DVC Singh as well as University Management and Dean of the Humanities Prof Maoto. Director of the School of Social Sciences Prof Sithole and the HOD Psychology Prof Sodi for supporting our research endeavours and the VC Prof Mokgalong.

Author details

Kathryn Nel* and Saraswathie Govender
University of Limpopo, Polokwane, South Africa

*Address all correspondence to: kathryn.nel@ul.ac.za

References

[1] Prien A, Grafe A, Rossler R, Junge A, Verhagen E. Epidemiology of head injuries focusing on concussions in team contact sports: A systematic review. Journal of Sports Medicine. 2018;**484**: 953-969. DOI: 10.1007/s40279-017-0854-4

[2] Janda DH, Bir CA, Cheney AL. An evaluation of the cumulative concussive effect of soccer heading in the youth population. Injury Control and Safety Promotion. 2002;**91**:25-31. DOI: 10.1076/icsp.9.1.25.3324

[3] Gardner A, Shores EA, Batchelor J. Reduced processing speed in Rugby Union players reporting three or more previous concussions. Archives of Clinical Neuropsychology. 2010;**253**: 174-181. DOI: 10.1093/arclin/acq007

[4] Maite P. Cumulative Mild Head Injuries in football (soccer): A comparison of cognitive deficit and post-concussive symptomology between University of Pretoria (AmaTuks) football players and University of Limpopo volleyball controls in South Africa [thesis]. Ga-Rankuwa, Pretoria: University of Limpopo (Medunsa Campus), South Africa; 2014

[5] Lezak MD, Howieson DB, Loring DW. Neuropsychological Assessment. 4th ed. New York, NY: Oxford University Press; 2004. DOI: 10.4236/jwarp.2018.101009

[6] Mureriwa JF. Traumatic brain injury and attention: Post-concussion symptoms and indices of reaction time [thesis]. Pretoria: University of South Africa; 1997

[7] Kolb B, Wishaw IQ. Fundamentals of Human Neurology. 5th ed. New York, NY: Worth Publishers; 2004. ISBN:10: 0716795868 2009

[8] Zillmer E, Spiers M, Culbertson WC. Principles of Neuropsychology. Belmont, CA: Thomson-Wadsworth; 2008. ISBN:10: 0-495-00376-X

[9] Nel C, Grace J, Nel K, Govender S. Cumulative mild head injury in schoolboy Rugby players. African Journal for Physical, Health Education, Recreation and Dance. 2015;**21**:92-102. ISSN: 1117-4315

[10] Finkelstein M. The scrum-down on brain damage effects of Cumulative Mild Head Injury in rugby a comparison of group mean scores between national rugby players and non-contact sport controls [thesis]. Grahamstown: Rhodes University; 1999

[11] Satz P, Alfano MS, Light R, Morgenstern H, Zaucha K, Asarnow RF, et al. Persistent post-concussive syndrome: A proposed methodology and literature review to determine the effects, if any, of mild head and other bodily injury. Journal of Clinical and Experimental Neuropsycholo Physician and Sportsmedicine gy. 1999;**215**: 620-628. DOI: 10.1076/jcen.21.5.620.870

[12] Binder LM, Rohling ML, Larrabee GJ. A review of mild head trauma. Part I: Meta-analytic review of neuropsychological studies. Journal of Clinical and Experimental Neuropsychology. 1997;**193**:421-431. DOI: 10.1080/01688639708403870

[13] Arciniegas DB, Anderson CA, Topkoff J, McAllister TW. Mild traumatic brain injury: A neuropsychiatric approach to diagnosis, evaluation, and treatment. Neuropsychiatric Disease and Treatment. 2005;**14**:311-327. PMC2424119

[14] Evans RW. The post-concussion syndrome. Neurology and General

Medicine. 1992;**104**:815-847. PMID: 1435659

[15] Rutherford A, Stephens R, Potter D, Fernie G. Neuropsychological impairment as a consequence of football (soccer) play and football heading: Preliminary analyses and report on university footballers. Journal of Clinical and Experimental Neuropsychology. 2005; **27**:299-319. DOI: 10.1080/13803390490515504

[16] Packard RC. Chronic post-traumatic headache: Associations with mild traumatic brain injury, concussion and post-concussive disorder. Current Pain and Headache Reports. 2008;**121**:67-73. PMID:18417027

[17] Silver J, McAllister T, Arciniegas D. Depression and cognitive complaints following mild traumatic brain injury. American Journal of Psychiatry. 2009; **1666**:653-661. DOI: 10.1176/appi.ajp.2009.08111676

[18] Echemendia RJ, Julian LJ. Mild traumatic brain injury in sports: Neuropsychology's contribution to a developing field. Neuropsychology Review. 2001;**112**:69-88. PMID: 11572472

[19] McCrory P, Meeuwisse W, Johnston K, Dvorak J, Aubry M, Molloy M, et al. Consensus statement on Concussion in Sport—The 3rd International Conference on Concussion in Sport held in Zurich, November 2008. Clinical Journal of Sports Medicine. 2009;**193**: 185-200. DOI: 10.1097/JSM.0b013e3181a501db

[20] Silver MJ, McAllister TW, Yudovsky MD. Mild brain injury and the post-concussion syndrome. In: Textbook of Traumatic Brain Injury. Arlington, VA: American Psychiatric Publishing, Inc; 2009. ISBN-10: 1585623571

[21] Cantu RC. Guidelines for return to contact sports after a cerebral concussion. Physician and Sportsmedicine. 1986;**1410**:75-83. DOI: 10.1080/00913847.1986.11709197

[22] Maroon JC, Lovell MR, Norwig J, Podell K, Powell JW, Hartl R. Cerebral concussion in athletes: Evaluation and neuropsychological testing. Neurosurgery. 2009;**473**:659-669. PMID: 10981755

[23] Aubry M, Cantu R, Dvorak J, Graf-Baumann T, Johnston K, Kelly J, et al. Summary and agreement statement of the first International Conference on Concussion in Sport, Vienna 2001. British Journal of Sports Medicine. 2002;**361**:6-10. PMID: 11867482

[24] Petchprapai N. Adaptation to mild traumatic brain injury among Thai adults [thesis]. Cleveland, Ohio: Case Western Reserve University; 2007

[25] Nell V, Brown DS. Epidemiology of traumatic brain injury in Johannesburg —II. Morbidity, mortality and aetiology. Social Science & Medicine. 1999;**333**: 289-296. PMID: 1925693

[26] Brain injury heads up for the cost of recovery [internet]. 2017. Available from: https://www.fanews.co.za/article/life-insurance/9/dread-disease-and-or-disability-critical-ilness/1085/brain-injuries-heads-up-for-the-costs-of-recovery/21948 [Accessed: 23.05.2018]

[27] Pope VJ, Edlow JA. Avoiding misdiagnosis in patients with neurological emergencies. Emergency Medicine International. 2012; ID 949275. DOI: 10.1155/2012/949275

[28] Mckee AC, Daneshvar D. The neuropathology of traumatic brain injury. Handbook of Clinical Neurology. 2015;**127**:45-66. DOI: 10.1016/B978-0-444-52892-6.00004-0

[29] Busl KM, Greer DM. Hypoxic-ischemic brain injury: Pathophysiology, neuropathology and mechanisms. NeuroRehabilitation. 2015;**26**:5-13. DOI: 10.3233/NRE-2010-0531

[30] Bey T, Ostick B. Second impact syndrome. The Western Journal of Emergency Medicine. 2009;**101**:6-10. PMID: 19561758

[31] Bigler ED. The lesion(s) in traumatic brain injury: Implications for clinical neuropsychology. Archives of Clinical Neuropsychology. 2001;**162**: 95-131. DOI: 10.1016/S0887-6177(00) 00095-0

[32] Strich SJ. Lesions in the cerebral hemispheres after blunt head injury. Journal of Clinical Pathology. 1970;**314**: 166-171. PMID: 4123922

[33] Niogi SN, Mukherjee P, Ghajar J, Johnson C, Kolster RA, Sarkar R, et al. Extent of microstructural white matter injury in post-concussive syndrome correlates with impaired cognitive reaction time: A 3T diffusion tensor imaging study of mild traumatic brain injury. American Journal of Neuroradiology. 2008;**295**:967-973. DOI: 0.3174/ajnr.A0970

[34] Daneshvar DH, O'Riley D, Nowinski CJ, McKee AC, Stern RA, Cantu RC. Long term consequences: Effects on normal development profile after concussion. Physical Medicine and Rehabilitation Clinics of North America. 2012;**224**:683-700. PMID: 22050943

[35] Medical coding reference [Internet]. 2018. Available from: https://www.icd10data.com/ [Accessed: 18.05.2018]

[36] Diagnostic and Statistical Manual of Mental Disorders—5th ed [Internet]. Available from: https://www.sciencetheearth.com/uploads/2/4/6/5/24658156/dsm-v-manual_pg490.pdf [Accessed: 04.06.2018]

[37] Carroll L, Cassidy JD, Peloso P, Borg J, von Holst H, Holm L, et al. Prognosis for mild traumatic brain injury: Results of the WHO collaborating centre task force on mild traumatic brain injury. Journal of Rehabilitation Medicine. 2004;**360**: 84-105. PMID: 15083873

[38] New Zealand Rugby League. New Zealand rugby league concussion policy [Internet]. Available from: http://websites.sportstg.com/get_file.cgi?id=1867985 [Accessed: 28.07.2018]

[39] Ruff T. Two decades of advances in understanding of Mild Traumatic Brain Injury. The Journal of Head Trauma Rehabilitation. 2001;**2005**:5-18. PMID: 15668567

[40] Paré N, Rabin LA, Fogel J, Pépin M. Mild traumatic brain injury and its sequelae: Characterisation of divided attention deficits. Neuropsychological Rehabilitation. 2009;**191**:110-137. DOI: 10.1080/09602010802106486

[41] Condor R, Condor AA. Neuropsychological and psychological rehabilitation interventions in refractory sport-related post-concussive syndrome. Brain Injury. 2014;**292**:1-14. DOI: 0.3109/02699052.2014.965209

[42] Boden BP, Tacchetti RL, Cantu RC, Knowles SB, Mueller FO. Catastrophic head injuries in high school and college football players. The American Journal of Sports Medicine. 2007;**357**: 1075-1081. DOI: 10.1177/0363546507 299239

[43] Carlson NE, Brenner LA, Wierman ME, Harrison-Felix C, Morey C, Gallagher S, et al. Hypogonadism on admission to acute rehabilitation is correlated with lower functional status at admission and discharge. Brain Injury. 2009;**234**:336-344. DOI: 10.1080/02699050902788535

[44] Tommasone BA, McLeod TVC. Contact sport concussion incidence. Journal of Athletic Training. 2006;**414**: 470-472. PMID: 17273475

[45] Zollman FS. Manual of Traumatic Brain Injury Management. 2nd ed. New York, NY: Demos Medical; 2016. ISBN 9781620700938

[46] A literature review on reaction time—Kosinki [internet]. 2012. Available from: https://www.semanticscholar.org/paper/A-Literature-Review-on-Reaction-Time-Kosinski/2cc72c884223f51be27e0e536d1fb19c1779f513 [Accessed: 25.04.2018]

[47] Ancer RL. Cumulative MHI in Rugby: Cognitive test profiles of professional Rugby and cricket players [thesis]. Grahamstown, South Africa: Rhodes University; 2000

[48] Ackermann TR. Minor "Dings"-Major Effects? A Study into the Cognitive Effects of Mild Head Injuries in High School Rugby. Grahamstown, South Africa: Rhodes University; 2001

[49] Partington-Nel K. Boys and Balls "skoppe en koppe" Cumulative Mild Head Injury in contact sport: An evaluation of the cognitive profile of adolescent rugby players compared with non-contact sport controls [mini-thesis]. Grahamstown, South Africa: Rhodes University; 2001

[50] Shuttleworth-Edwards AB, Noakes TD, Radloff SE, Whitefield VJ, Clark SB, Roberts CO, et al. The comparative incidence of reported concussions presenting for follow-up management in south African Rugby union. Clinical Journal of Sport Medicine. 2008;**185**: 403-409. DOI: 10.1097/JSM.0b013e3181895910

[51] Faber J, Fonseca LM. How small sample size influences research outcomes. Dental Press Journal of Orthodontics. 2014;**19**:27-29. PMCID: PMC4296634

[52] Nel K, Govender S, Rapetsoa M, Nel C. Cumulative mild head injury (CMHI) among college rugby players. A replication and extension study. Journal of Psychology in Africa. 2017;**276**: 549-552. DOI: 10.1080/14330237.2017.1399571

[53] Rizi RM, Yeung SS, Stewart NJ, Yeung EW. Risk factors that predict severe injuries in university rugby sevens. Journal of Science and Medicine in Sport. 2017;**20**:648-652. DOI: 10.10.16/j.sams.2016.11.022

[54] Leung FT, Smith MMF, Brown M, Rahmann A, Mendis MD, Hides JA. Epidemiology in Australian school level rugby union. Journal of Science and Medicine in Sport. 2017;**20**:740-744. DOI: 10.1016/j.sa,s.2017.3.006

[55] Archbold HAP, Rankin AT, Webb M, Nicholas R, Eames NWA, Wilson RK, et al. Recurrent injury patterns in adolescent rugby. Physical Therapy in Sport. 2018;**33**:12-17. DOI: 10.1016/j.ptsp.2018.06.005

[56] Ahmed OH, Hall EE. It was only a mild concussion: Exploring the description of sports concussion in online news articles. Physical Therapy in Sport. 2018;**23**:7-13. DOI: 10.1016/j.ptsp.2016.07.003

[57] Kosoy J, Feinstein MD. Evaluation and management of concussion in young athletes. Current Problems in Pediatric and Adolescent Health Care. 2018;**48**:1-11. DOI: 10.1016/j.cppeds.2018.06.002

[58] Tysvaer AT, Storli OV, Bachen NI. Soccer injuries to the brain. A neurologic and electroencephalographic study of former players. Acta Neurologica Scandinavica. 1989;**802**:151-156. DOI: 10.1177/036354658901700421

[59] Barnes BC, Cooper L, Kirkendall DT, McDermott TP, Jordan BD, Garrett WE. Concussion history in elite male and female soccer players. The American Journal of Sports Medicine. 1998;**263**:433-438. DOI: 10.1177/03635465980260031601

[60] Kross R, Ohler K, Barolin GS. Effects of heading in soccer on the head—A quantifying study of soccer players. EEG-EMG Zeitschrift fur Elektroenzephalograhie Elektromyographie und Verwandte Gebiete. 1986;**144**:209-212. PMID: 6418516

[61] Abreau F, Templer DI, Schuyler BA, Hutchison HT. Neuropsychological assessment of soccer players. Neuropsychology. 1990;**43**:175-181. DOI: 10.1037/0894-4105.4.3.175

[62] Putukian M, Echemendia RJ, Mackin S. The acute neuropsychological effects of heading in soccer: A pilot study. Clinical Journal of Sport Medicine. 2000;**102**:104-109. PMID: 10798791

[63] Kirkendall DT, Garrett WE. Heading in soccer: Integral skill or grounds for cognitive dysfunction? Journal of Athletic Training. 2001;**363**: 328-333. PMID: 12937505

[64] Maite P, Nel K, Govender S. Reaction time deficits incurred by cumulative mild head injury (CMHI) and post-concussion symptoms (PCS) between contact and non-contact sports players. A prospective study. Journal of Psychology in Africa. 2017;**266**:555-557. DOI: 10.1080/14330237.2016.1250415

[65] Nordstrom A, Nordstrom P, Ekstrand J. Sports-related concussion increases the risk of subsequent injury by about 50% in elite male football players. British Journal of Sports Medicine. 2014;**48**:1447-1450. DOI: 10.1136/BKS[PRTS-2013-093406

[66] Reilly T. Energetics of high-intensity exercise (soccer) with particular reference to fatigue. Journal of Sports Sciences. 1989;**153**:257-263. DOI: 10.1080/026404197367263

[67] Should young soccer players be banned from heading the ball. 2016. Available from: https://www.theguardian.com/sport/2016/jan/22/us-young-soccer-players-heading-ball [Accessed: 05.05.2018]

[68] Hammami N, Hattabi S, Salhi A, Rezgui T, Oueslati M, Bouassida A. Combat sports injuries profile: A review. Science & Sports. 2018;**33**:73-79. DOI: 101016/j.scispo.2017.04.014

[69] Mohotti D, Fernando PLN, Zaghoul A. Evaluation of possible head injuries ensuing a cricket ball impact. Computer Methods and Programmes in Biomedicine. 2018;**158**:193-205. DOI: 10.101016/j.cmpb.2018.02.2017

[70] Tripathi M, Shukla DP, Bhat DI, Bhagavatula ID, Mishra T. Craniofacial injuries in professional cricket: No more a red herring. Neurosurgical Focus. 2016;**40**:1-11. DOI: 10.317/2016.2FOCUS15341

[71] Jordan BD. Chronic traumatic brain injury in boxing. Seminars in Neurology. 2000;**20**:179-185. DOI: 10.4085/1062-6050.52.2.05

[72] Bentz JE. Concussion in American football and sports. Available from: http://www.jlgh.org/JLGH/media/Journal-LGH-Media-Library/Past%20Issues/Volume%208%20-%20Issue%203/bentz8_3.pdf [Accessed: 31.07.2018]

[73] Izraelski J. Concussions in the NHL: A narrative review of the literature. Journal of the Canadian Chiropractic Association. 2014;**58**:346-352. PCMID: PMC4262814

Chapter 4

Neuronal and Glial Biomarkers Research for Traumatic Brain Injury

Alexander Rodríguez, Eliana Cervera and Pedro Villalba

Abstract

The potential of early neurological inaccurate assessment of severity in patients with traumatic brain injury (TBI) has been highlighted; in some cases, for example, the severity of the injury is overestimated or underestimated. These findings have led to the search of biomarkers associated with early brain injury. Research in this field has exponentially increased over the past 20 years, with most publications on the subject in the last 10 years, whose results range from promising findings to other sometimes inconclusive one. An ideal biomarker should be able to demonstrate high sensitivity and specificity for brain injury, among other aspects. Literature has shown that there is not a single biomarker that predicts the patient's clinical decline with high sensitivity and specificity. Instead, it is required to use a panel of markers that reflect different aspects of head trauma. This chapter gives a review of the most promising biomarkers studied as predictors of severity of TBI, with a special focus on their nature, location, basal concentrations, and methods by which they can be quantified in blood samples.

Keywords: acute brain injury, biomarkers, blood-brain barrier, prognosis, Glasgow Coma Scale

1. Introduction

Every year, 1.1 million Americans are treated in emergency rooms for traumatic brain injury (TBI): 235,000 are hospitalized for nonfatal TBI and 50,000 died. In Finland, a prospective study found that 3.8% of the population had experienced at least one hospitalization due to traumatic brain injury before 35 years of age. Similarly, another study in New Zealand found that at 25 years of age, 31.6% of the population had experienced at least one TBI that required medical attention (hospitalization, emergency department, or doctor's office). It is estimated that 43.3% of Americans have residual disability 1 year after the damage. The most recent estimate of the prevalence of the US civilian residents living with disability after hospitalization with TBI is 3.2 million [1].

TBI is assessed and classified clinically according to the Glasgow Coma Scale (GCS) [2] and by imaging: axial computed tomography (CT) and magnetic resonance imaging (MRI). However, the use of GCS as a diagnostic tool is subject to important limitations, and it is difficult to assess the eye opening in patients with serious lesions on the face; likewise, the verbal response cannot be correctly estimated in individuals who are under the influence of psychoactive drugs and/or alcohol, and in those who are intubated or sedated will have limited linguistic capacities [3]. Given that the severity of the neurological injury may be underestimated in some cases and overestimated in others, attention has been focused on early assessment strategies in patients with TBI and their inaccuracy in special and frequent circumstances [4].

In view of the high rate of intubation and difficulties in the proper evaluation of the eye opening, Stocchetti et al. concluded that motor GCS score was more important than eye opening or verbal responses to predict the severity of the neurological injury. Other recent research has provided evidence that the use of sedative drugs avoids the accurate assessment of GCS during the first 24 h [5].

Other challenges for diagnosis are presented by the progressive nature of some brain injuries, which can lead to further neurological deterioration. In addition, neurological responses after TBI may vary over time for reasons unrelated to the injury. For example, trauma is frequently associated with alcohol and drug intoxication [6]. These factors together place the GCS in a position full of limitations that diminish its reliability as a highly sensitive test in specific and not infrequent circumstances such as those already mentioned.

On the other hand, neuroimaging techniques are used to provide objective information about the injury and its location [7] and are not influenced by the aforementioned confounding factors. However, the CT scan has a low sensitivity for diffuse brain injury, when the TBI is mild [8] and the availability and usefulness of MRI in the acute stage is limited. These facts, among others, have led to the search for alternative methods to assess the damage, being of special interest, the search for biomarkers, which are more reliable indicators of neuronal injury, due to its molecular context and its early expression.

Research in this field has increased exponentially in the last 20 years, with most publications on the subject in the last 10 years. Most markers are associated with cell damage. **Table 1** presents a summary of the TBI biomarkers most studied to date, including information about their nature, tissue location, molecular weight, half-life, basal levels, and physiopathological significance.

The main physiopathological mechanisms reflected by the glial or neuronal biomarkers are the disruption of the blood-brain barrier (BBBD) and neuronal injury, respectively. Taking into account this basis, it would be advantageous to have a panel of complementary biomarkers that show different temporal profiles and that reflect different physiopathological conditions subsequent to TBI. In a parallel manner, Papa et al. [9] propose that an ideal biomarker should have the following characteristics:

1. demonstrate high sensitivity and specificity for brain injury;
2. stratify the patients according to the severity of the injury;
3. have rapid appearance in the accessible biological liquid;
4. provide information about injury mechanisms;
5. have biokinetic properties;
6. monitor the progress of the disease and the response to the treatment;
7. predict the functional result; and
8. easily measured by simple techniques widely available.

Biomarker	Location	Molecular mass [KDa]	Nature	Half life	Basal concentrations	Significance
UCH-L1	Neuronal	20 [41] 24 [42]	Ubiquitination enzyme	20 minutes [43]	0.12 ng/mL [44]	Neuronal injury
NSE	Neuronal	90 [45] 78 [46]	Enzyme	24 h [46] 48 h [41]	<12.5 ng/mL [47] ≤15 ng/mL [46]	Neuronal injury
αII-espectrina	Neuronal	280 [41]	Cytoskeleton component protein	2.9 h [48]	—	Apoptosis
SBDP		120 [41]		1.5 days [49]		
		145 [41]		1 day [49]		
		150 [41]		1 day [49]		
S-100B	Glial (astrocytes)	21 [50]	Calcium binding protein	97 minutes [47] 112 minutes [43]	0.328–0.01 pg/mL [11]	BBBD
MBP	Glial (oligodendrocytes and Schwann cells)	18.5 [50]	Myelin sheath component protein	12 h [43]	<0.3 ng/mL [50]	White matter injury
GFAP	Glial (astrocytes)	40–53 [30]	Cytoskeleton component protein	—	<0.03 ng/mL [30]	BBBD and neuronal injury

Table 1.
Main biomarkers in TBI and their properties.

In this chapter, we present a compendium of the most studied biomarkers in the TBI, its possible applications, and the current techniques for its detection.

2. Most studied biomarkers in TBI

As explained in previous paragraphs, there is no single biomarker that is sufficiently sensitive and specific to study the physiopathological mechanisms that derive from head trauma. Next, we will mention some of the most studied biomarkers given its rapid elevation after trauma and its relationship with the mechanism of injury. One of the most studied biomarkers is the Ca binder protein S-100β, a glial protein at the astrocyte level that is related to alterations in the blood-brain barrier [10]. Its rapid elevation and its considerable concentration release in the serum facilitate the study of the protein and its correlation with the severity of the injury. Due to the type of cells found in the central nervous system, it is necessary to study biomarkers that allow us to demonstrate not only glial injury but also neuronal. One of the most studied biomarkers in this sense is the C-terminal hydrolase of ubiquitin-L1, which is a highly specific cytoplasmic neuronal enzyme [11, 12]. Finally, we will delve into glial fibrillary acidic protein (GFAP), which is also a glial protein and is part of the cytoskeleton of astrocytes and is also related to the disruption of the blood-brain barrier [11, 13].

2.1 The Ca binder protein S-100β

S-100 β is a central nervous system (CNS) protein found predominantly in astrocytes and is the most studied peripheral biomarker of BBBD. This calcium binding protein (CBP) S-100β increases initially after the accident and then decreases rapidly after the traumatic injuries. In cell models, their release has been demonstrated from the first 15 seconds after the trauma. In humans, the earliest that has been detected is 30 minutes posttrauma. The approximate half-life of this protein is 97 minutes [10], the peak occurs on day 0, and the concentrations decrease toward the sixth day in both CSF and serum.

Goyal et al. [14] reported basal levels of S-100β in healthy CSF controls of 0.0754–0.0034 ng/mL and in serum of 0.328–0.101 pg/mL. This protein has been studied extensively in mild TBI (mTBI), so that high levels in serum are associated with an increase in the incidence of post-concussion syndrome [15] and neurological dysfunction. There are also several studies that have reported a correlation between serum levels of S-100β and the presence of pathological findings in cerebral magnetic resonance imaging (MRI), as well as abnormalities in neuropsychological exploration after mTBI [16].

Most studies show that the S-100β measurement can distinguish injured patients from noninjured patients with an uncertain degree of utility in predicting mortality either acutely or at several points in time (**Table 2**) [17–19]. In general terms, S-100β is a sensitive but not specific predictor of CT abnormalities. Using low serum cut-off values, the sensitivity oscillates between 90 and 100% with a specificity between 4 and 65%.

Müller et al. [17] reported a sensitivity of 0.95 (95% CI 0.76–1.0) for S-100β measured within the first 12 h with a specificity of 31% (95% CI 0.25–0.38) relative to abnormal findings on skull CT scan in a study of 226 adult patients admitted to the hospital with a diagnosis of mild TBI (GCS 13–15). Biberthaler et al. [19] found similar results using a cut-off level of S-100β of 0.1 ng/mL, measured within the first 3 h posttrauma in 1309 patients with mTBI and correlating them to head CT findings. The sensitivity was 99% (95% CI 0.96–1.0), and the specificity was 30% (95% CI 0.29–0.31).

Reference	Detection method	Sample	Findings
Goyal et al. [14]	ELISA	CSF and serum	Increase in CSF and serum first 6 days post-trauma Correlation between serum and CSF levels decreased over time Level in CSF is a potential predictor of GOS and DRS Mean and peak are predictors of mortality in severe TBI
Berger et al [51]	Automated LIAISON system [AB DiaSorin, Bromma, Sweden]	Serum	Significantly elevated in intracranial injury It cannot replace the clinical examination or the use of CT in mTBI It can serve as support for the selection of patients for TC S: 90–100%, E: 4–65%
Biberthaler et al [19]	Elecsys S100 [Roche Diagnostics, Mannheim, Germany]	Serum	Increase was related to findings in the CT scan S: 99%, E: 30%
Biberthaler et al [52]	Long term and Rapid test	Serum	Concentrations were significantly correlated using the two measurement techniques; cut-off value calculated: 0.18 ng/mL. S: 100%, E: 46%
Bazarian, et al [21]	ELISA	Serum	S: 80%, E: 40%

Table 2.
Summary of the evidence reported in the literature on biomarkers in S-100B.

The usefulness of S-100β as a marker does not seem to be affected by the concomitant consumption of alcohol. Mussack et al. conducted a study in which they included patients with mild TBI with demonstrated blood alcohol levels (mean = 182 mg/dL), and found that the sensitivity of S-100β in the first 3 h posttrauma was 100% (95% CI 0.83 a 1.0) and the specificity was 50% (95% CI 0.41–0.59) [20].

On the other hand, Bazarian et al. studied 96 patients with TBI, GCS 13–15 who also presented trauma of extracranial localization, and found a sensitivity of 80% (95% CI 0.36–0.96) and a specificity of 40% (95% CI 0.01–0.09) for S-100β with a cut-off value of 0.08 ng/mL [21].

From the studies described above, it can be deduced that the sensitivity increases as the time elapsed between the trauma and the sample taking (window) decreases, as well as an increase in specificity is observed when the cut-off value increases. In contrast, the limitations of the use of S-100β as a marker are due to the marked decrease in sensitivity and specificity in the context of the polytraumatized patient, since the presence of concomitant extracranial trauma also causes the release and plasma elevation of this protein. The presence of S-100β has been reported in tissues other than the nervous one, mainly in adipose tissue [22]. From this observation, a negative effect on the specificity of this marker is expected, due to the increase that would occur in the context of extracranial lesions, as occurs in the polytraumatized patient.

Pham et al. [22] characterized the tissue specificity of S-100β and evaluated the extracranial sources of this marker and how they affect serum levels of this marker. For this purpose, they performed the extraction of proteins from nine different human tissues (liver, bladder, kidney, colon, lung, muscle, pancreas, adipose tissue, brain, tonsils, stomach, and skin) and their subsequent analysis through ELISA and Western blot in 200 subjects receiving chemotherapy for the management of CNS lymphomas. A dose of mannitol (1.4M) was administered intra-arterially in the carotid or vertebral artery, subsequently confirming the presence of BBBD by a head CT performed immediately after chemotherapy.

The results presented in that study showed that extracranial sources of S-100β do not affect serum levels. Therefore, the diagnostic value and the negative predictive value of S-100β are not compromised in the context of patients with neurological diseases, but without traumatic lesions, whether cerebral or extracranial.

Goyal et al. [14] also evaluated S-100β as a prognostic biomarker in adult subjects with severe TBI (sTBI) by comparing the results with the S-100β temporal profiles in both CSF ($n = 138$ subjects) and serum ($n = 80$ subjects) for 6 days. The variables used to evaluate the extracerebral sources of S-100β in serum were: long bone fracture, Injury Severity Score (ISS), and isolated skull trauma. After TBI, levels of S-100β in CSF and serum were increased compared to healthy controls during the first 6 days after TBI ($p \leq 0.005$ and $p \leq 0.031$). Although levels in CSF and serum had a high correlation at the early post-TCE time points, this association decreased with time. The bivariate analysis showed that subjects who had temporary CSF profiles with higher concentrations of S-100B had higher acute mortality ($p < 0.001$) and worse Glasgow Outcome Scale (GOS; $p = 0.002$) and disability scores (DRS) ($p = 0.039$) 6 months after the injury. Temporary profiles in serum were associated with acute mortality ($p = 0.015$), possibly as a result of the extracerebral sources of S-100β in the serum, represented by high ISSs ($p = 0.032$).

Due to its temporal elevation profile, and the pathophysiological mechanisms that cause its release toward serum, S-100β constitutes an excellent candidate as an early biomarker of TBI, with the possible limitation in patients with concomitant trauma in other sites that leads to the serum elevation of S-100β from extracranial sources.

2.2 Ubiquitin C-terminal hydrolase-L1 (UCH-L1)

The C-terminal hydrolase of ubiquitin-L1 (ubiquitin C-terminal hydrolase-L1, UCH-L1) is an E2 conjugation enzyme present in the cytoplasm of almost all neurons [13] and has previously been used as a neuronal histological marker due to its great abundance and specific expression in these cells [11]. Its location has also been shown in neurons of the peripheral nervous system, particularly in the neuromuscular junction [12], as well as in cells of the neuroendocrine system. In addition, the presence of UCH-L1 has been demonstrated in aortic endothelial cells and in smooth muscle and tumor cells [23]. This enzyme accomplishes the function of adding and removing ubiquitin from proteins in order to promote its degradation via the proteasome-dependent pathway [24].

UCH-L1 is one of the most recent biomarkers proposed for TBI, and for this reason, there are still limited data that demonstrate its usefulness (**Table 3**).

Three isoenzymes of UCH (UCH-L1, UCH-L2, and UCH-L3) have been identified, being UCH-L1, the only one present in high concentrations in the central nervous system [24]. In a prospective case-control study with 66 patients, Papa et al. [24] obtained ventricular CSF samples for each patient after 6, 12, 24, 48, 72, 96, 120, 144, and 168 h after TBI for the UCH-L1 detection by ELISA. The severity was determined by the Glasgow Scale (GCS) and CT findings. Mortality and neurological sequelae were evaluated at 6 months. This study showed that patients with TBI had a significant elevation of CSF UCH-L1 levels at each point in time compared to controls, with total mean in TBI patients = 44.2 ng/mL (±7.9) vs. 2.7 ng/mL (±0.7) in controls ($p < 0.001$). Significantly elevated levels of UCH-L1 were found in

Reference	Detection method	Sample	Findings
Papa et al. [24]	ELISA	CSF	Increase at 6, 12, 24, 48, 72, 96, 120, 144, and 168 h post-trauma, X = 44.2 ng/mL (±7.9), versus controls X = 2.7 ng/mL (±0.7) ($p < 0.001$). Also elevated when it exists: lower GCS at 24 h, post-trauma complications, deaths in the first 6 weeks, or serious sequelae at 6 months.
Brophy et al. [53]	ELISA	CSF and serum	Significant correlation between biokinetics and means of (UCH-L1) in CSF and serum in severe TBI (rs = 0.59, $p < 0.001$) (AUC, rs = 0.3, p = 0.027). Increased levels <24 h posttrauma, statistically significant in Cmax (0–24 h) in CSF and serum in those who died.
Mondello et al. [26]	Sandwich ELISA	CSF and serum	It remains elevated up to 7 days after TBI, serum AUC and statistically significant CSF at all-time points up to 24 h ($p < 0.001$). Levels in <12 h in GCS 3–5 > GCS 6–8 (p = 0.07 and p = 0.02, Mann-Whitney test, respectively). Significantly higher and prolonged serum and CSF levels in non-survivors. A level of >5.22 ng/mL was a predictor of mortality (OR 4.8).
Papa et al. [11]	ELISA	Serum	Elevated in GCS 15 vs. controls without trauma (AUC 0.8) and controls with trauma. Higher elevation in GCS 15 plus TAC or neurosurgical intervention requirement. It provides evidence as a potential marker of mild TBI.
Kou et al. [27]	Electrochemiluminescence immunoassay (ECL-IA)	Serum	Complements brain MRI in the detection of injury. Significantly elevated levels in patients in the acute state of mild TBI.
Diaz-Arrastia et al. [28]	Sandwich ELISA	Serum	Measurement <24 h posttrauma distinguished presence and absence of intracranial lesions (AUC of 0.713). No correlation between levels in mild TCE and recovery at 6 months. Significant increase in levels in moderate/severe TCE compared with mild TBI. Good sensitivity to discriminate between TCE and controls (AUC 0.87). Combination with GFAP showed greater sensitivity and specificity for the diagnosis of TBI (AUC 0.94).
Puvenna et al. [15]	ELISA	Serum	There were no significant differences between the levels of negative controls and TCE <6 h posttrauma, independent of the CT. The levels were high after each game but without correlation with the number of hits received.

Table 3.
Summary of the evidence reported in the literature on UCH-L1.

patients with a lower score in the GCS at 24 h, in those who had presented post-trauma complications, in those who died within the first 6 weeks, and in those with severe sequelae at 6 months. These data suggest that this marker would be useful in determining severity in patients with TBI. Similar studies with larger samples are required to validate these findings.

Additional studies have confirmed the positive correlation between the concentrations of UCH-L1 at the CSF level and serum samples [25]. Similarly, Mondello et al. [26] conducted a case-control study with 95 patients with severe TBI in order to evaluate the CSF and serum concentrations of UCH-L1 by sandwich ELISA and its association with clinical results. The temporal profile of the marker in both CSF and serum was studied during the first 7 days following the trauma and compared with controls showing significantly higher levels compared to the controls throughout the 7-day period, also confirming a high sensitivity and specificity for the diagnosis of TBI versus controls, with statistically significant serum AUC and CSF values at all-time points up to 24 h ($p < 0.001$).

The levels of UCH-L1 in the first 12 h in both CSF and serum in patients with GCS 3–5 were also significantly higher than in those with GCS 6–8. In addition, UCH-L1 levels in CSF and serum appeared to distinguish between patients with severe TBI survivors and nonsurvivors within the study, such that those who died had significantly higher CSF and serum UCHL1 levels, as well as greater permanence of these levels over time. In this study, a serum level of UCH-L1 > 5.22 ng/mL was a predictor of mortality (OR 4.8).

Papa et al. [11] also analyzed UCH-L1 in serum taken in the first 4 h posttrauma in patients with mild (n = 86) and moderate (n = 10) TBI, as well as in controls with trauma and controls without trauma. For patients with a GCS of 15, serum UCH-L1 was significantly elevated compared to controls without trauma, with an AUC of 0.87, and was also compared with controls with trauma, and was even higher in those patients with GCS of 15 who also had positive findings on the CT scan or required some neurosurgical intervention, suggesting that UCH-L1 may be a potential marker of mild TBI. Additionally, 5% of patients with GCS of 15 (4/77) required neurosurgical intervention, which was higher than the 1% found in patients with GCS 14–15 reported in the study by Jagoda et al., in which the samples were taken within the first 24 h posttrauma [10].

It is inferred from these data that the earlier it is detected posttrauma, the sensitivity of this marker increases. In a smaller study (n = 9), serum UCHL1 (taken <6 h posttraumatic) was found to be significantly elevated in patients with mild TBI [27].

In another study focused on all levels of severity of TBI, serum UCH-1 measured before 24 h posttrauma could distinguish patients with intracranial lesions from those without intracranial lesions with an AUC = 0.713 [28]. However, there was no correlation between UCH-L1 levels in patients with mTBI and recovery at 6 months as measured by the GOSE scale. While there was a significant increase in UCH-L1 levels in patients with moderate/severe TBI compared to mild TBI, patients with mild TBI were not compared with controls.

In a research carried out in a secondary school, Puvenna et al. [15] selected 15 American football players; they obtained serum samples before and after each of two different games. They did not observe significant differences between the levels of UCH-L1 between the negative controls and the positive individuals for mild TBI within the first 6 h posttrauma, regardless of whether or not positive CT findings existed. In addition to this, there was no correlation between the serum levels of UCH-L1 and the number of impacts received. The levels of UCH-L1 and S-100β, markers of neuronal injury and BBBD, respectively, were both elevated after each game. However, only S-100β, unlike UCH-L1, was correlated with the number of hits received and the UCH-L1 elevation did not correlate with the S-100β increments. The authors suggest that elevated postgame UCH-L1 levels may be due to the release of this protein from the neuromuscular junction.

It can be concluded that there are very divergent data regarding the use of UCH-L1 as a serum biomarker of mild TBI. Some studies suggest that it is a promising marker, while others do not find a correlation with the lesion. Release from sources other than the central nervous system could contribute to elevated serum levels.

2.3 The fibrillary acid glial protein (GFAP)

Glial fibrillary acidic protein (GFAP) is a protein derived from glial cells, which is a part of the intermediate filament of the cytoskeleton of astrocytes, where it is the most abundant protein. It is considered a specific marker of CNS diseases, and is also related to several neuronal processes' harmful agents that compromise the integrity of the blood-brain barrier [29], and has been shown to be a potentially useful biomarker for predicting clinical outcomes in TBI. Its normal level in serum is <0.03 ng/mL [30], so any elevation thereof will indicate BBBD (**Table 4**).

Due to its great immunoreactivity, GAFP has been used as an indicator of brain injury in experimental models of mTCE [31]. The first successful measurement of GFAP in human blood was made in 1999 in 12 of 25 patients with severe TBI [32]. Using a weight drop model with mice [33] to evaluate two levels of mTBI, one with hemorrhage (complicated mTBI) and another without bleeding (uncomplicated mTBI), Yang et al. [34] found that serum GFAP was significantly elevated in both injury models at 90 minutes and 6 h after injury, but had returned to normal at 24 h.

In the study of Kou et al. [27], significantly elevated serum levels of GFAP in the first 24 h posttrauma in 9 mTBI patients was also reported; this elevation being even more significant in those with hemorrhagic lesions; however, the small size of the sample does not allow the conclusions to be validated.

In another study, Mondello et al. [35] evaluated whether the relationship between a neuronal marker (UCH-L1) and a glial marker (GFAP) correlates with the presence of different intracranial pathologies after brain trauma. They obtained serum samples from 59 patients with sTBI on admission to the hospital and measured levels of UCH-L1 and GFAP. The glial/neuronal ratio (GNR) was measured as the quotient between the concentrations of GFAP and UCH-L1. Logistic regression analysis identified variables associated with the type of injury. The increase in GNR was associated independently with the type of injury, but not with the age, gender, GCS, or trauma mechanism. This quotient was significantly higher in the patients who died, but it was not an independent predictor of mortality. The GNR had a median of 0.85 and correlated positively with age.

When evaluating the CT scan of the skull on admission, 29 patients presented a diffuse lesion and 30 localized lesions. The GNR was significantly higher in the group with focal lesions compared to the group with diffuse lesions. The receiver operating characteristic (ROC) analysis showed that the GNR discriminated between the two types of injury. GNR was more accurate when performed early than when it was done late (**Table 4**).

These data indicate that the GNR provides valuable information about the different types of injury, which is of great clinical utility. In addition, the GNR can help to identify the pathophysiological mechanisms subsequent to the different types of TBI. This is very useful when implementing therapeutic measures.

In an investigation carried out by Papa et al. [36], the capacity of the GFAP taken <4 h posttrauma was compared to predict intracranial lesions in the CT compared to S-100β. Although patients had GCS 9–15, only 3 of 209 patients had GCS <13 and only 10% had intracranial lesions, both S-100β and GFAP were significantly elevated in all patients, and even more so in those with intracranial lesions. For those patients with GCS 14–15, the AUC for the identification of intracranial lesions was 0.82 for GFAP and 0.77 for S-100β.

In the presence of extracranial lesions and using a cut-off value of 0.067 ng/mL, GFAP was 100% sensitive and 55% specific in the prediction of intracranial lesions. With a cut-off value of 0.20 ng/mL, S-100β also had 100% sensitivity but only 5% specificity. This study concludes that GFAP exceeds S-100β in the identification of intracranial lesions in mild and moderate TBI, even in the presence of extracranial lesions.

Reference	Detection method	Sample	Findings
Kou et al. [27]	Electrochemiluminescence immunoassay (ECL-IA)	Serum	Significantly elevated in all cases of intracranial hemorrhage, with potential screening capacity. Small size of the sample does not allow to validate the conclusions.
Mondello et al. [35]	Sandwich ELISA	Serum	Evaluation of GNR (GFAP/UCH-L1): Median = 0.85, positive correlation with age (R = 0.45, p = 0.003). Greater in focalized lesions vs. diffuse lesion (1.77 vs. 0.48, respectively, p = 0.003). Different type of lesions (AUC = 0.72, p = 0.003). More precise early measurement (<12 h posttrauma) vs. late (AUC = 0.80, p = 0.002). Independent association with the type of injury, but not with the GCS. Independent predictor of mortality.
Papa et al. [36]	ELISA	Serum	S-100B and GFAP significantly elevated in all patients, especially in intracranial injuries. For GCS 14–15, AUC = 0.82 in identification of intracranial lesions for GFAP (0.77 for S-100B). With extracranial lesions and cut-off 0.067 ng/mL, GFAP: S = 100% and E = 55% to predict intracranial lesions. GFAP outperforms S-100B in the identification of intracranial lesions in mild and moderate TBI, even in the presence of extracranial lesions.
Papa et al. [54]	ELISA	Serum	GFAP-BDP significantly elevated in mild TCE vs. controls with or without trauma. AUC = 0.88 to identify brain injury in GCS 15. Higher levels in GCS 15 with positive CT.
Okonkwo et al. [55]	ELISA	Serum	GFAP-BDP <24 h posttrauma distinguished between mild and moderate/severe TBI (AUC of 0.87). Controls were not included, mild to moderate TCE was not compared, and most of the statistical analysis was made with all levels of severity at the time.

Table 4.
Summary of the evidence reported in the literature on GFAP in TBI.

In general, GFAP seems to increase in TBI and could represent a more sensitive marker than S-100β for the identification of intracranial lesions. However, for further validation, more studies are needed that focus specifically on mTBI (GCS 13–15), which include appropriate controls and adequate statistical comparisons.

3. Discussions and conclusions

One of the main purposes of the search for potential biomarkers in the TBI is to predict the presence of pathological findings in head CT and brain MRI; however, the studies published in this regard are inconclusive, and the evidence favors the use of S-100β over other markers in mTBI, as a predictor of negative-CT.

For example, Posti et al. [37] showed that patients with orthopedic trauma had higher levels of GFAP at admission, than those with mTBI and negative-CT (p = 0.026), and did not show that UCH-L1 levels presented significant differences in both groups, performing measurements at different time points, which suggest that these markers are not useful for distinguishing patients with negative-CT mTBI from patients with orthopedic trauma, and that high levels of UCH-L1 or GFAP can lead to a false diagnosis of mTBI in polytraumatized patients, leading to the unnecessary use of neuroimaging.

On the other hand, the use of the S-100β marker has been recommended in the Scandinavian guidelines for the initial management of minimal, mild, and moderate head injuries in adults [38] as an alternative to reduce the number of CT in the subgroup of mTBI with low risk of intracranial complications or surgical interventions. More studies are needed that show the usefulness of S-100β as a predictor of neurodeterioration in moderate TBI.

The use of neuroimaging is necessary to improve the accuracy of biomarkers in the diagnosis and prognosis of patients who have suffered a TBI, with CT being the first option and the one with the most studies in relation to the release and correlation of biomarkers. Some reviews report higher serum S-100β levels in more severe, focal lesions, compared to diffuse lesions using Marshall scale, and a strong correlation between S100B increasing and the severity of the CT finding when using the sum of Rotterdam CT score and Stockholm CT score [54].

Olivecrona et al. reported how S-100β and neuronal specific enolase (NSE) levels correlate with CT findings using the aforementioned scales. Specifically, S-100β levels, but not to the NSE levels, correlates with Morris-Marshall score for the classification of traumatic subarachnoid hemorrhage (tSAH). This is probably associated with the physiopathological pathways described by each of these biomarkers after a neurotrauma. Likewise, the volume of the parenchymal contusions is also associated with the S-100β levels. Furthermore, in mild TBI, initial low levels of S-100β can be used as a predictor of a stationary injury, suggesting that the CT classification does not evolve [55].

Diagnosis of severity and prognosis of CT findings cannot be performed by a single biomarker test. Instead, a combination of biomarkers of diverse origins and pathways displays a better performance. Thereby, the joint use of GFAP, heart fatty acid binding protein (H-FABP), S-100β, and IL-10 results in a more efficient diagnostic tool with a 46% specificity and 100% sensitivity for predicting CT injuries. This biomarker panel increases specificity by 14% compared to the best single biomarker [56].

The ALERT-TBI study, developed in 22 centers in USA and Europe, validated the ability of the combination of UCH-L1 and GFAP to predict CT injuries within 12 h of mTBI, resulting in a sensitivity of 97.6%, a negative predictive value (NPV) of 99.6%, and a specificity of 36.4%. Therefore, when indicating CT only in those patients with a positive GFAP and UCH-L1 test, the CT use could be reduced by approximately one-third. The extent of these findings to patients with moderate TBI is uncertain [57].

The study of the available evidence on the different serum markers in TBI presented in this chapter allows us to conclude that, currently, there is not a single biomarker capable of predicting the clinical deterioration of patients with high sensitivity and specificity. However, the pathophysiological mechanisms of TBI suggest that instead, a panel of markers that reflect different aspects of traumatic injury should be available, including BBBD and neuronal injury.

The literature has shown that the joint use of S-100β and GFAP or UCH-L1 would represent a valuable early prognostic and follow-up tool in TBI in addition to the GCS and the CT, thus guiding the decisions of initial management and aggressive interventions.

Likewise, given that the kinetic profile of these markers is different, since it presents peaks of appearance earlier than others and different times of permanence in serum, its usefulness would also be correlated with different post-traumatic stages, so that S-100β and UCH-L1 are better early markers [24, 25], whereas GFAP is a better predictor of CT lesions and surgical interventions in the first 7 days post-trauma in mild and moderate TBI [27].

In addition to the above, the literature also shows that these biomarkers are being measured with techniques that demand the use of complex equipment and procedures (such as ELISA) in which the use of labels is necessary [6, 39], displaying the need for the development of rapid and cost-effective techniques that allow the implementation of biomarkers in the clinical setting.

Acknowledgements

We thank Universidad del Norte and Colciencias for the financial support of the research project in which the development of this work is framed.

Conflict of interest

The authors declare no conflict of interest.

Author details

Alexander Rodríguez*, Eliana Cervera and Pedro Villalba
Department of Medicine, Universidad del Norte, Barranquilla, Colombia

*Address all correspondence to: alexandersanjuan@uninorte.edu.co

References

[1] Corrigan J, Selassie A, Orman J. The epidemiology of traumatic brain injury. The Journal of Head Trauma Rehabilitation. 2010;**2**(2):72-80. DOI: 10.1097/HTR.0b013e3181ccc8b4

[2] Matis G, Birbilis T. The Glasgow coma scale—A brief review past, present, future. Acta Neurologica Belgica. 2008;**108**(3):75-89

[3] Forastero P, Echevarria C, Barrera J. Traumatismos craneoencefálicos. Escalas de valoración para la medida de resultados en rehabilitación. Rehabilitación. 2002;**36**(6):408-417. DOI: 10.1016/S0048-7120(02)73314-8

[4] Stocchetti N et al. Inaccurate early assessment of neurological severity in head injury. Journal of Neurotrauma. 2004;**21**(9):1131-1140. DOI: 10.1089/neu.2004.21.1131

[5] Livingston B, Mackenzie S, MacKirdy F, Howie J. Should the presedation glasgow coma scale value be used when calculating acute physiology and chronic health evaluation scores for sedated patients? Critical Care Medicine. 2000;**28**(2):389-394

[6] Mondello S, Muller U, Jeromin A, Streeter J, Hayes R, Wang K. Blood-based diagnostics of traumatic brain injuries. Expert Review of Molecular Diagnostics. 2011;**11**(1):65-78. DOI: 10.1586/erm.10.104

[7] Carney N et al. Guidelines for the management of severe traumatic brain injury, fourth edition. Journal of Neurotrauma. 2017;**80**(1):6-15. DOI: 10.1227/NEU.0000000000001432

[8] Zhang J, Puvenna V, Janigro D. Biomarkers of traumatic brain injury and their relationship to pathology. In: Laskowitz D, Grant G, editors. Translational Research in Traumatic Brain Injury. Boca Raton, FL: CRC Press/Taylor and Francis Group; 2016. pp. 263-276. DOI: 10.1201/b18959-13

[9] Papa L et al. Use of biomarkers for diagnosis and management of traumatic brain injury patients. Expert Opinion on Medical Diagnostics. 2008;**2**(8):937-945. DOI: 10.1517/17530059.2.8.937

[10] Jagoda A et al. Clinical policy: Neuroimaging and decisionmaking in adult mild traumatic brain injury in the acute setting. Annals of Emergency Medicine. 2008;**52**(6):714-748. DOI: 10.1016/j.annemergmed.2008.08.021

[11] Papa L et al. Serum levels of ubiquitin C-terminal hydrolase distinguish mild traumatic brain injury from trauma controls and are elevated in mild and moderate traumatic brain injury patients with intracranial lesions and neurosurgical intervention. Journal of Trauma and Acute Care Surgery. 2012;**72**(5):1335-1344. DOI: 10.1097/TA.0b013e3182491e3d

[12] Chen F, Sugiura Y, Myers K, Liu Y, Lin W. Ubiquitin carboxyl-terminal hydrolase L1 is required for maintaining the structure and function of the neuromuscular junction. Proceedings of the National Academy of Sciences of the United States of America. 2010;**107**(4):1636-1641. DOI: 10.1073/pnas.0911516107

[13] Bishop P, Rocca D, Henley J. Ubiquitin C-terminal hydrolase L1 (UCH-L1): Structure , distribution and roles in brain function and dysfunction. The Biochemical Journal. 2016;**473**(16):2453-2462. DOI: 10.1042/BCJ20160082

[14] Goyal A et al. S100b as a prognostic biomarker in outcome prediction for patients with severe traumatic brain injury. Journal of Neurotrauma. 2013;**30**(11):946-957. DOI: 10.1089/neu.2012.2579

[15] Puvenna V et al. Significance of ubiquitin carboxy terminal hydrolase L1 elevations in athletes after subconcussive head hits. PLoS One. 2014;**9**(5):e96296. DOI: 10.1371/journal.pone.0096296

[16] Adrian H et al. Biomarkers of traumatic brain injury: Temporal changes in body fluids. eNeuro. 2016;**3**(6):ENEURO.0294-16.2016. DOI: 10.1523/ENEURO.0294-16.2016

[17] Müller K et al. S100B serum level predicts computed tomography findings after minor head injury. The Journal of Trauma. 2007;**62**(6):1452-1456. DOI: 10.1097/TA.0b013e318047bfaa

[18] Ingebrigtsen T et al. The clinical value of serum S-100 protein measurements in minor head injury: A Scandinavian multicentre study. Brain Injury. 2000;**14**(12):1047-1055

[19] Biberthaler P et al. Serum S100B concentration provides additional information for the indication of computed tomography in patients after minor head injury: A prospective multicenter study. Shock. 2006;**25**(5):446-453. DOI: 10.1097/01.shk.0000209534.61058.35

[20] Mussack T et al. Immediate S-100B and neuron-specific enolase plasma measurements for rapid evaluation of primary brain damage in alcohol-intoxicated, minor head-injured patients. Shock. 2002;**18**(5):395-400

[21] Bazarian J, Beck C, Blyth B, Von Ahsen N, Hasselblatt M. Impact of creatine kinase correction on the predictive value of S-100B after mild traumatic brain injury. Restorative Neurology and Neuroscience. 2010;**24**(3):163-172

[22] Pham et al. Extracranial sources of S100B do not affect serum levels. PLoS One. 2010;**5**(9):e12691. DOI: 10.1371/journal.pone.0012691

[23] Campbell L, Thomas J, Lamps L, Smoller B, Folpe A. Protein gene product 9.5 (PGP 9.5) is not a specific marker of neural and nerve sheath tumors: An immunohistochemical study of 95 mesenchymal neoplasms. Modern Pathology. 2003;**16**(10):963-969. DOI: 10.1097/01.MP.0000087088.88280.B0

[24] Papa et al. Ubiquitin C-terminal hydrolase is a novel biomarker in humans for severe traumatic brain injury. Critical Care Medicine. 2010;**38**(1):138-144. DOI: 10.1097/CCM.0b013e3181b788a

[25] Brophy G et al. Biokinetic analysis of ubiquitin C-terminal hydrolase-L1 (UCH-L1) in severe traumatic brain injury patient biofluids. Journal of Neurotrauma. 2001;**28**(6):861-870. DOI: 10.1089/neu.2010.156

[26] Mondello S et al. Clinical utility of serum levels of ubiquitin C-terminal hydrolase as a biomarker for severe traumatic brain injury. Neurosurgery. 2012;**70**(3):666-675. DOI: 10.1227/NEU.0b013e318236a809

[27] Kou Z et al. Combining biochemical and imaging markers to improve diagnosis and characterization of mild traumatic brain injury in the acute setting: Results from a pilot study. PLoS One. 2013;**19**(8):11, e80296. DOI: 10.1371/journal.pone.0080296

[28] Diaz-Arrastia et al. Acute biomarkers of traumatic brain injury: Relationship between plasma levels of ubiquitin C-terminal hydrolase-L1 and glial fibrillary acidic protein. Journal of Neurotrauma. 2014;**31**(1):19-25. DOI: 10.1089/neu.2013.3040

[29] Eng L, Ghirnikar R, Lee Y. Glial fibrillary acidic protein: GFAP-thirty-one years (1969-2000). Neurochemical Research. 2000;**25**(9):1439-1451

[30] Ingebrigtsen T, Romner B. Biochemical serum markers of

traumatic brain injury. The Journal of Trauma. 2002;**52**(4):798-808

[31] Saatman K, Bolton A. Regional neurodegeneration and gliosis are amplified by mild traumatic brain injury repeated at {24-hour} intervals. Journal of Neuropathology and Experimental Neurology. 2014;**73**(10):933-947. DOI: 10.1097/NEN.0000000000000115

[32] Missler U, Wiesmann M, Wittmann G, Magerkurth O, Hagenström H. Measurement of glial fibrillary acidic protein in human blood: Analytical method and preliminary clinical results. Clinical Chemistry. 1999;**45**(1):138-141

[33] Albert-Weissenberger C, Sirén AL. Experimental traumatic brain injury. Experimental & Translational Stroke Medicine. 2010;**2**(1):16

[34] Yang S et al. A murine model of mild traumatic brain injury exhibiting cognitive and motor deficits. The Journal of Surgical Research. 2013;**184**(2):981-988. DOI: 10.1186/2040-7378-2-16

[35] Mondello S et al. Glial neuronal ratio: A novel index for differentiating injury type in patients with severe traumatic brain injury. Journal of Neurotrauma. 2012;**29**(6):1096-1104. DOI: 10.1089/neu.2011.2092

[36] Papa L et al. GFAP out-performs S100beta in detecting traumatic intracranial lesions on computed tomography in trauma patients with mild traumatic brain injury and those with extracranial lesions. Journal of Neurotrauma. 2014;**31**(22):1815-1822. DOI: 10.1089/neu.2013.3245

[37] Posti JP et al. Glial fibrillary acidic protein and ubiquitin C-terminal hydrolase-L1 are not specific biomarkers for mild CT-negative traumatic brain injury. Journal of Neurotrauma. 2017. DOI: 10.1089/neu.2016.4442

[38] Undén L et al. Validation of the Scandinavian guidelines for initial management ofminimal, mild and moderate traumatic brain injury in adults. BMC Medicine. 2015;**13**:292. DOI: 10.1186/s12916-015-0533-y

[39] Strathmann FG et al. Blood-based biomarkers for traumatic brain injury: Evaluation of research approaches, available methods and potential utility from the clinician and clinical laboratory perspectives. Clinical Biochemistry. 2014;**47**(10-11):876-888. DOI: 10.1016/j.clinbiochem.2014.01.028

[40] Papa L, Brophy G, Welch R, Lewis L, Braga C, Tan C, et al. Time course and diagnostic accuracy of glial and neuronal blood biomarkers GFAP and UCH-L1 in a large cohort of trauma patients with and without mild traumatic brain injury. JAMA Neurology. 2016;**73**(5):551-560. DOI: 10.1001/jamaneurol.2016.0039

[41] Kövesdi E, Lückl J, Bukovics P, Farkas O, Pál J, Czeiter E, et al. Update on protein biomarkers in traumatic brain injury with emphasis on clinical use in adults and pediatrics. Acta Neurochirurgica. 2010;**152**:1-17. DOI: 10.1007/s00701-009-0463-6

[42] North S, Shriver-Lake L, Taitt C, Ligler F. Rapid analytical methods for on-site triage for traumatic brain injury. Annual Review of Analytical Chemistry. 2012;**5**(1):35-56. DOI: 10.1146/annurev-anchem-062011-143105

[43] Mondello S, Akinyi L, Buki A, Robicsek S, Gabrielli A, Tepas J, et al. NIH public access. 2013;**70**(3):666-675

[44] Benito I, Rodríguez J. Determinación radioinmunométrica de la enolasa neuronal específica en humor acuoso y suero, en pacientes con retinoblastoma. Revista Española de Medicina Nuclear e Imagen Molecular. 2000;**7**:472-478

[45] Test ID: NSESF. Neuron-Specific Enolase (NSE), Spinal Fluid [Internet]. 2018. Available from: https://www.mayocliniclabs.com/test-catalog/pod/MayoTestCatalog-Rochester-LaboratoryReferenceEdition-SortedByTestName-duplex.pdf [Accessed: 7 December 2018]

[46] Dash P, Zhao J, Hergenroeder G, Moore A. Biomarkers for the diagnosis, prognosis, and evaluation of treatment efficacy for traumatic brain injury. Neurotherapeutics. 2010;**7**(1):100-114. DOI: 10.1016/j.nurt.2009.10.019

[47] Wang K, Posmantur R, Nath R, McGinnis K, Whitton M, Talanian R, et al. Simultaneous degradation of alphaII and betaII-spectrin by caspase 3 (CPP32) in apoptotic cells. The Journal of Biological Chemistry. 1998;**273**(35):22490-22497

[48] Brophy G, Pineda J, Papa L, Lewis S, Valadka A, Hannay H, et al. alphaII-Spectrin breakdown product cerebrospinal fluid exposure metrics suggest differences in cellular injury mechanisms after severe traumatic brain injury. Journal of Neurotrauma. 2009;**26**(4):471-479. DOI: 10.1089/neu.2008.0657

[49] Berger R, Hymel K, Gao W. The use of biomarkers after inflicted traumatic brain injury: Insight into Etiology, pathophysiology, and biochemistry. Clinical Pediatric Emergency Medicine. 2006;**7**(3):186-193. DOI: 10.1016/j.cpem.2006.06.001

[50] Biberthaler P, Mussack T, Wiedemann E, Kanz K-G, Mutschler W, Linsenmaier U, et al. Rapid identification of high-risk patients after minor head trauma (MHT) by assessment of S-100β: Ascertainment of a cut-off level. European Journal of Medical Research. 2002;**7**(4):164-170

[51] Brophy G, Mondello S, Papa L, Robicsek S, Gabrielli A, Tepas J, et al. Biokinetic analysis of ubiquitin C-terminal hydrolase-L1 (UCH-L1) in severe traumatic brain injury pa¬tient biofluids. Journal of Neurotrauma. 2011;**28**(6):861-870. DOI: 10.1089/neu.2010.1564

[52] Papa L, Lewis L, Falk J, Zhang SS, Giordano P, et al. Elevated levels of serum glial fibrillary acidic protein breakdown products in mild and moderate traumatic brain injury are associated with intracranial lesions and neurosurgical intervention. Annals of Emergency Medicine. 2012;**59**:471-483. DOI: 10.1016/j.annemergmed.2011.08.021

[53] Okonkwo D, Yue J, Puccio A, Panczykowski D, Inoue T, Mcmahon P, et al. GFAP-BDP as an acute diagnostic marker in traumatic brain injury: Results from the pros¬pective transforming research and clinical knowledge in traumatic brain injury study. Journal of Neurotrauma. 2013;**30**(17):1490-1497. DOI: 10.1089/neu.2013.2883

[54] Thelin E et al. A review of the clinical utility of serum S100B protein levels in the assessment of traumatic brain injury. Acta Neurochirurgica. 2017;**159**(2):209-225. DOI: 10.1007/s00701-016-3046-3

[55] Olivecrona Z et al. Association of ICP, CPP, CT findings and S-100B and NSE in severe traumatic head injury. Prognostic value of the biomarkers. Brain Injury. 2014:29. DOI: 10.3109/02699052.2014.989403

[56] Lagerstedt L, Egea-Guerrero JJ, Bustamante A, Rodríguez-Rodríguez A, El Rahal A, Quintana-Diaz M, et al. Combining H-FABP and GFAP increases the capacity to differentiate between CT-positive and CT-negative patients with mild traumatic brain injury. PLoS One. 2018;**13**(7):e0200394. DOI: 10.1371/journal.pone.0200394

[57] Bazarian JJ, Biberthaler P, Welch RD, Lewis LM, Barzo P, Bogner-Flatz V, et al. Serum GFAP and UCH-L1 for prediction of absence of intracranial injuries on head CT (ALERT-TBI): A multicentre observational study. Lancet Neurology. 2018;**17**(9):782-789. DOI: 10.1016/S1474-4422(18)30231-X

Section 3

Treatment and Multiple Therapeutic Strategies

Chapter 5

Use of Neuroprotective agents for Traumatic Brain Injury

Mohammad Meshkini, Ali Meshkini and Homayoun Sadeghi-Bazargani

Abstract

Traumatic brain injury (TBI) is the leading cause of mortality and morbidity especially in young ages, while over 30 years of neuroprotective agents use for TBI management provided neither any recommended agent for favorable outcome nor less adverse effects in TBI management yet. This review got selected keywords' search and ran in known international and local databases, with no limitation up to September 6, 2015. Related to the subject, clinical human studies have been selected for the review. Data from 32 studies were classified into 10 subgroups. About 18 studies with a population of 4637 participants were included in 6 topic reviews and meta-analyses. Oxygen use in acute management of TBI to reduce mortality rates could be recommended. Corticosteroid use in solo acute TBI management is prohibited due to increasing risk of mortalities. However, in dual-diagnosed patients (TBI and spinal cord injury (SCI) together), corticosteroid use should be obtained by a Bracken protocol. The use of citicoline in acute TBI is no more supported. The use of cyclosporine-A for ICP control depends on the resources and physician's decision. Rivastigmine use for chronic neurocognitive conditions of TBI management had some beneficence in severely impaired participants. However, the use of other agents in TBI has no field of support yet.

Keywords: traumatic brain injury, head injury, neuroprotective agents, systematic review, meta-analysis

1. Introduction

1.1 Description of the condition

Traumatic brain injury (TBI), which is also known as head injury [1–3], is the leading cause of mortality and morbidity [1, 4–6], especially in young ages [1]; that is defined as "the occurrence of injury to the head, that is, associated with symptoms or signs attributable to the injury such as decreased level of consciousness, amnesia, other neurological or neuropsychological abnormalities, skull fracture, intracranial lesions or death." [6].

Epidemiological studies, demonstrate following statements in USA [4];

- The incidence rate of 558 cases per 100,000 person each year,
- TBI related disability estimated as 33 new cases per 100,000 people in a year,
- More than 50,000 deaths each year,
- Motor vehicle collisions (MVC) is the responsible for 50% of TBI causes, following by falls (38%), and violence (also including attempted suicide) 4%,
- TBI costs more than $48 billion a year. About 2.5 and 6.5 million Americans alive today have had a TBI assault. "Survivors of TBI are often left with significant cognitive, behavioral, and communicative disabilities" [7]. According to the chronology period and the state of the condition, it categorizes under "Primary" and "Secondary" injury [1].

1.2 Description of the intervention

According to medical subheadings (MeSH) definition, Neuroprotective agents are "Drugs intended to prevent damage to the brain or spinal cord from ischemia, stroke, convulsions, or trauma. Some must be administered before the event, but others may be effective for some time after. They act by a variety of mechanisms, but often directly or indirectly minimize the damage produced by endogenous excitatory amino acids" [8]. As mentioned in the MeSH definition, there are variety of drugs and their action mechanisms to minimize the TBI damage; the breadth list of trials on www.clinicaltrial.gov for "Neuroprotective Agents" and "Traumatic Brain Injury" terms, states this. A recent study of Burns et al. declared 30 years of using Neuroprotective agents on animal models forecasting the same effect on humans failed, and represents to use animal models as new cases for stem cell studies as well, rather than formerly known for using Neuroprotective agents [9], which is confirmed by other studies too [10, 11].

The recent challenging review and meta-analyses study of Leucht et al. about efficacy of commonly used major drugs for medical and psychological conditions, seems to be a practice-challenging article for all physicians over the world [12]; this meta-analyzed article's results on major commonly used drugs showed the small to medium effect of 13 drugs and nearly medium to favorable effect of 3 drugs out of 19 major commonly used drugs for variety of clinical or mental conditions; collecting these information together rings a bell; how to use the most effective interventions for conditions?

2. Literature review

There are wide variety of Neuroprotective agents, and breadth studies on human and animal cases, the following lists the agents which were studied on human clinical trials:

2.1 Oxygen

The vital element of life and viability of neurons. Hypoxia leads to anaerobic metabolism, acidosis, and reduction in cellular metabolism. Neurons messaging conduction ability disturbs due to loss of their ability to maintain ionic homeostasis.

Free oxygen radicals also accumulate and degrade cell membrane; which all if lead to irreversible changes in neuron cells, it "results in unavoidable cell death." There are also Cochrane reviews for hyperbaric oxygen (HBO_2) and hyperventilation (NBH) use in TBI [1, 2].

2.2 Corticosteroids

Inflammatory process after TBI, which causes brain edema and intracranial pressure (ICP) rise, performed the hypothesis of using corticosteroids for TBI, the primary researches and studies showed the beneficial effect of this intervention, while CRASH trial in 2005 and an updated Cochrane review after that, challenged the efficacy of corticosteroids use for TBI [4]; further from this study's proposal, steroids using for spinal cord injury (SCI) seems to have beneficial effects; also there is a Cochrane review for its neuroprotection beneficence in SCI assaults [13].

2.3 Progesterone

It has a wide variety of neuroprotection mechanisms of action, as an antioxidant agent, by reducing brain edema and inflammatory-related factors, controlling of vasogenic edema through blood brain barrier (BBB) reconstitution and aquaporin-4 water transporter modulation, axonal regenerating stimulant, inhibition of inflammatory cytokines production, synaptogenesis and dendritic arborization, altering glutamate receptor activity to reduce excitotoxicity of injury and also taking all these effects by its receptor's key rolling [14–16]. Also inhibition of ion flux cell pores like L-type calcium channel, potassium, and sodium voltage-gates, as well GABA-A receptors, all result in vasoconstriction and reducing edema that seem likely to dihydropyridine's mechanism of action, without its side effects like dizziness, peripheral edema, hypotension, reflex tachycardia and headaches [17, 18].

2.4 Monoaminergic agents

Amphetamine and other promotors of neuroaminergic neurotransmission have been suggested to improve the functional recovery of the brain after TBI. There is also a Cochrane review for these agents [19].

2.5 Erythropoietin (EPO)

A glycoprotein hormone of cytokine type-I super family, that its anti-apoptotic and anti-inflammatory properties, also interaction of EPO with neural voltage-gated calcium channels, and EPO with EPO-receptors increasing of local production after TBI, seems to be EPO's mechanisms of action [20–22].

2.6 Magnesium sulfate and other magnesium salts

Reduction in serum magnesium levels after TBI, and beneficial effects of magnesium therapy in animal models, conceptualized its use for human cases, its failure in recent studies, came to the conclusion of blood brain barrier (BBB) effect on this agent's transmission [23].

2.7 Cerebrolysin

"Cerebrolysin is a peptide-preparation, produced by the bio-technologically standardized enzymatic breakdown of purified porcine brain proteins." mechanism of action is not fully understood, but animal studies, suggest improved neuronal oxygen utilization, reduction of cerebral lactic acid concentration and free oxygen radical concentrations [24].

2.8 Citicoline (CDP-choline) and other cholinergics

Adenosine tri-phosphate (ATP) is responsible for cell membrane sodium-potassium (Na-K) ATPase pump's function; TBI related cell membrane un-integrity and accumulation of extracellular water, leads to the known brain edema, also formation of lipid peroxidase. Cholinergic agents' effects in cell-oxygenation cycles and formation of ATP indirectly may cause cell wall integrity formation as well as prevent further secondary injuries [25].

2.9 NeuroAid

A Chinese medicine, also known as MCL601 and MCL901 (a.k.a. Simplified to NeuroAid or NeuroAid-II, respectively), which showed Neuroprotective effects in stroke trials [26, 27].

2.10 Cyclosporine A (CsA)

Preservation of mitochondrial function after TBI is the recommended mechanism of action for this agent [28, 29].

2.11 Rivastigmine

Mostly known for its cholinesterase inhibitory (ChE-inh) effects, that improves cholinergic function of brain in Alzheimer disease (AD) trials; there are also TBI trials based on hypothesis of post-traumatic cholinergic deficiencies [30, 31].

2.12 Piracetam

This intervention seems to improve neurocognitive state of patients without any remarkable effects on the mortalities.

2.13 Anti-epileptic drugs

Anti-epileptic drugs may have some Neuroprotective effects as well, but they are not included in this study, however these drugs have their own Cochrane review [3].

2.14 Why it is important to do this review?

The review, been performed on Neuroprotective agents for TBI, fulfill the systematic review & analysis on each one of the mentioned agents in "Literature Review" section of this study; "Drug data is complex and requires thoughtful consideration regarding which medication and therapies are best suited for certain situation and patients." Leucht et al. declared [12]. Burns et al. work didn't clearly demonstrate the use of new stem cell studies on TBI, but it has hopes for SCI [9]. Studies showed people may not feel comfortable with stem cell therapies because of "don't want to get the risk of cancer" or "don't want to have another surgery" who also are about 58–63% of patients [9] that may lead our current hopes to neuroprotective use, despite stem cells.

3. Methods

Criteria for considering studies for this review.

3.1 Types of studies

The back-bone of present study's meta-analyses made by including RCTs, which their reporting quality, compared to CONsolidated Standards Of Reporting Trials (CONSORT-statement) 2010 (http://www.consort-statement.org/); other related to subject articles, with good and qualitative methods in reporting, included according to the study's statistical consultant's point of view. Guidelines or protocols, letter to editors and systematic reviews are excluded from the data analyses.

3.2 Types of participants

Humans of any age, and with any severity (mild, moderate, severe) of focal or diffuse TBI, have been included; neither animal studies nor pre-clinical (in-vivo) trials included in this study.

3.3 Types of interventions

The related studies about the mentioned agents in "Literature Review" section with any frequency, any chronicity and any mode of use.

3.4 Types of outcome measures

Outcomes were analyzed in two main groups for acute TBI management:

3.4.1 Primary outcomes

- Mortality and vegetative state
- Good recovery and mild disability

As measured by Glasgow Outcome Scale (GOS) or Extended Type (GOS-E) after 3–6 months of patient follow-up; severe disabilities weren't included in the analyses.

3.4.2 Secondary outcomes

- Any adverse effects or events of interventions during the trial.

For chronic TBI management, outcomes were mostly analyzed for neurocognitive state.

3.5 Search methods for identification of studies

The search strategy was not restricted by language, date, participants race, gender or publication status; but date limitation implemented to the referencing databases (i.e., SCOPUS and Thomson Reuters Web of Science) for after 2000 search results, also limiting results to human studies where possible.

3.5.1 Electronic searches

The web-based searched data-bases are:

- Cochrane CENTRAL (September 6, 2015)
- MedLine through PUBMED (September 6, 2015)
- SCOPUS (September 6, 2015)
- Thomson Reuters Web of Science (September 6, 2015)
- SID.ir (September 6, 2015)
- Barekat Knowledge Deployment Foundation (formerly known as IRAN-MEDEX) (September 6, 2015)
- ClinicalTrials.gov (September 6, 2015).

3.5.2 Searching other resources

Other related articles, came out through Internet search for full-text articles, and full-text requests through www.researchgate.net, and skimming in bibliographies of articles. Also contacting with experts to enrich the including data.

3.6 Data collection and analysis

Zotero v.4.0.28 (available from www.zotero.org) was used as Reference Manager of this review, while Cochrane's Review Manager (RevMan v5.3) taken the role of meta-analyses and conducting the whole study as well.

3.7 Selection of studies

Screening of related articles via their titles and abstracts done by two review authors (AM and MM); further assessment of including articles obtained by applying CONSORT-statement 2010 on full-texts of the articles by two review authors (HSB and MM), also disagreements of the screening-phase articles and the decision to include non-RCT studies referred to statistical consultant of study (HSB). The Preferred Reporting Items for Systematic Reviews & Meta-Analyses (PRISMA) statement, lead authors to diagram the process of study-selection (**Figure 1**).

3.8 Data extraction and management

Two review authors (AM and MM) extracted data from the included studies using CONSORT 2010 characteristics; any disagreements, referred to the third author (HSB).

3.9 Assessment of risk of bias in included studies

Two review authors (HSB and MM) assessed RCTs using the "risk of bias" assessment tool of "Cochrane Handbook for Systematic Reviews of Interventions v. 5.1.0" [32].

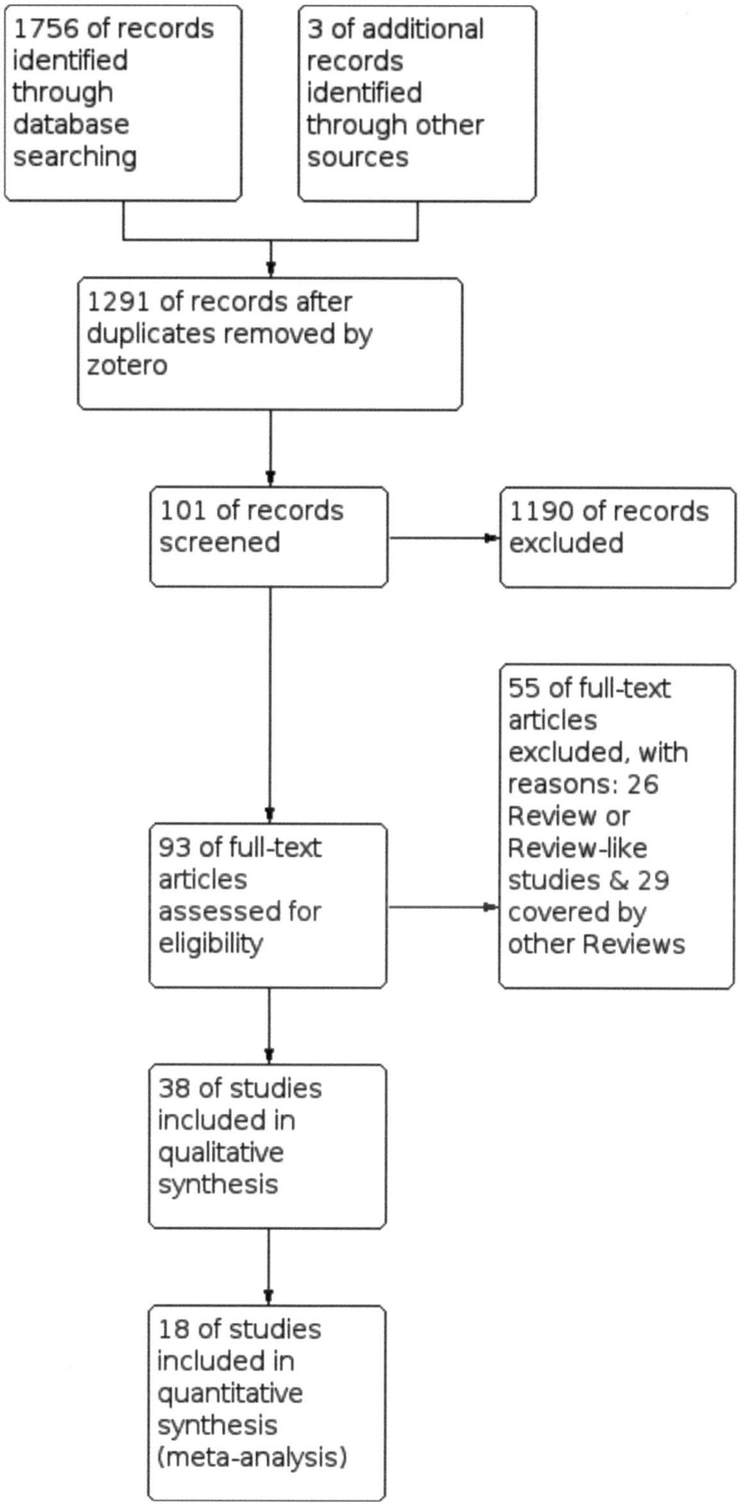

Figure 1.
PRISMA template (study flowchart).

3.10 Measures of treatment effect

Glasgow Outcome Scale (GOS) or its Extended type used as the assessment tool for severe TBIs outcome, considered to take place in the analyses; otherwise, patients preference of interventions [i.e., patient reported outcome (PRO)] in studies' results, were taken as outcome measurements of included studies in mild and moderate TBIs. More information of each intervention outcome analysis is represented under "Results" section of the study.

3.11 Unite of analysis issues

All meta-analyses of fixed effects model for dichotomous quantitative results, done by their risk ratio and confidence interval (CI) = 95%; continuous data results analyzed by their mean difference and CI = 95%; random effects model applied if $I^2 > 50\%$ [33].

3.12 Dealing with missing data

According to search strategy, authors have to conclude as possible as the available studies for the review, reduce selection and information biases as well; but some data would never been available even after contacting the original investigators or correspondence authors; the authors strategy for dealing with these kind of missing data was to ignore the missing data and to analyze only the available data, but if it's assumed that the missing data, had a huge effect on the analysis, in the HSB's point of view, using statistical models to allow missing data in analysis, making assumptions about their relationships with the available data were taken, fortunately there was no such conflict during this study's process.

3.13 Assessment of heterogeneity

Any heterogeneity of studies referred to HSB, for statistical consultant's point of view to reassess their use in the study, if they didn't have the availability to take part in study, they had been excluded.

3.14 Assessment of reporting biases

Probable reporting biases of studies, reported by using "Cochrane Handbook for Systematic Reviews of Interventions v. 5.1.0" method [32].

3.15 Subgroup analysis and investigation of heterogeneity

Data analyses based on:

- Favorable outcome of intervention (mostly based on GOS or GOS-E);
- Mortality and vegetative-state analysis
- Probable side-effects of interventions.

If some interesting results of study(ies) are brought, they'd be analyzed separately.

3.16 Sensitivity analysis

All of the search studies results reporting, were based on significant meaningful of results with $p < 0.05$ and CI = 95%.

4. Results

4.1 Description of studies

Qualitative report of study results, was completed with RCTs meta-analyses. Which from 38 RCTs included in this study, 18 RCTs been meta-analyzed. Also previous review papers in this field covered RCTs which are not included in this review again, i.e., 27 of these RCTs were discussed by Alderson et al. Cochrane review of corticosteroids [4]; Monoaminergic agents Cochrane review by Forsyth et al. covered 20 of them [19]. However previously discussed papers in HBO_2 and NBH Cochrane reviews, didn't take part in this review again [1, 2], which limited oxygen topic's studies to seven papers and no new articles found for those other two topics; **Figure 1** and **Table 1** summarize the finding information. The 18 included meta-analyzed studies, have a population of 4637 patients, of which 3650 patients were for four new phase-III RCTs altogether. Furthermore information is available under each topic of "Results of the search" section.

4.2 Results of the search

4.2.1 Oxygen

This intervention is the most eligible one of all other experimental trials of TBI neuroprotectives. Two Cochrane reviews were conducted under the title

Neuroprotective	Total no. RCTs	No. RCTs in this study	No. RCTs included	No. acute TBI RCTs	No. chronic TBI RCTs	Studies populations	No. phase-3 RCTs
Oxygen	24	7	4	1	3	205	0
Corticosteroid	27	All study results from Alderson 2006 Cochrane review [4]					
Progesterone	7	7	4	4	–	2320	2
Monoaminergics	20	All study results from Forsyth 2011 Cochrane review [19]					
Erythropoietin	4	4	2	2	–	645	1
Magnesium	4	1	Vink et al. [23] results combined with this pilot study				0
Cerebrolysin	1	1	1	1	–	32	0
Citicoline	4	4	4	3	1	1196	1
NeuroAid	0	0	0	0	0	0	0
Cyclosporine A	5	5	2	2	–	89	0
Rivastigmine	3	3	1	–	1	157	0
Piracetam	3	0	0	unknown	unknown	unknown	unknown
Miscellaneous	unknown	6	0	–	–	–	–
Total	**102**	**38**	**18**	**13**	**5**	**4637**	**4**

Table 1.
Neuroprotective RCTs for TBI at a glance.

"Hyperventilation therapy for acute traumatic brain injury (Review)," which established in 1997 and continued till the last updated paper of 2009 [2], and "Hyperbaric Oxygen therapy for the adjunctive treatment of traumatic brain injury (Review)," which started from 2004 and was last revised in 2012 [1]. These reviews demonstrated reduction in mortality rates while using oxygen in TBI, but there was no adequate evidences to support better clinical outcomes. This review's search results got eight more new additional studies. One observational study to investigate guideline adherence about pre-hospital advanced airway attempt for oxygenation in 54 severe TBI patients, that resulted in good adherence of performers to the guidelines [34], which also reported in other studies aimed to assess practitioners' adherence to guidelines, even better if they were supported by strong evidences [35, 36], but not satisfied results which recommended revision for guidelines; and seven clinical trials, mostly case-sham control design method, that five of them were pilot phase-II studies supported by Department of Defense/Veteran Affair (DoD/VA) for a huge phase-III RCT on HBO_2 use [37–41], the other two trials were Rockswold et al. and Boussi-Gross et al. for combined HBO_2/NBH treatment and HBO_2 in a case control and cross-over method trials respectively [42, 43]. Except than Rockswold et al. study on acute TBI patients, other studies' participants were of chronic impaired TBI patients.

Overall patients analyses without loss to follow-ups are 205 patients as 48 in Wolf et al., 42 in Rockswald et al., 56 in Boussi-Gross et al. and 59 in Cifu et al.; This review, include all of these trials in narrative review, but because of their heterogeneity in reporting outcomes, no meta-analysis conducted for the results [37, 40, 42, 43].

The only study reported mortality was Rockswold et al. for 16% in HBO_2/NBH combined group and 42% in control group, that might be due to its acute phase design for TBI management [43] in comparison to other three trials were about mild chronic TBI management. Boussi-Gross et al. study reports significant improvements in cognitive states (memory, attention, executive function, information processing speed) of patients with mild TBI in chronic phase, while DoD/VA related studies didn't state any significant changes of cognitive functions between HBO_2 and sham-control groups according to their Immediate Post Concussion Assessment and Cognitive Testing (ImPACT) and Post-Traumatic Stress Disorder Check List-Military (PCL-M) assessment tools [37, 40, 42]; Rockswald et al. acute phase study's GOS outcome for HBO_2/NBH combined group, demonstrated significant improvements ($p = 0.024$), and better outcomes for cerebral metabolism, partial oxygen pressure in brain and ICP [43].

Also only side-effect report was in Wolf et al. study that ear barotrauma and headache were the most common conditions [41], while Cifu et al. study on eye tracking abnormalities didn't demonstrate any significantly meaningful improvements for HBO_2 treatment participants, Wolf et al. results on Snellen chart assessment of visual acuity showed improvements in both HBO_2 and Sham-control groups (22 of 47 eyes and 25 of 46 eyes respectively), also reduction of visual acuity was less in the sham-control group (6 of 47 eyes and 3 of 46 eyes) [39, 41].

4.2.2 Corticosteroids

Cochrane updated review for corticosteroids in 2006, recommended no more trials of corticosteroids for TBI according to phase-III CRASH trial's results, another update of this review at January 7, 2009, found no novel study to investigate. There was no more study in current review's search results too.

4.2.3 Progesterone

The 2012 Cochrane review of "Progesterone for acute traumatic brain injury (Review)," based on three phase-II trials, declared that it would be updated as two more multi-centric clinical trials' results came out [5]; at the time of current review's searching for Neuroprotective agents, those mentioned trials and one more study been achieved [10, 11, 44]. Authors complete reading each one of the studies by comparing them to CONSORT 2010 checklist, finally included four studies [10, 11, 45, 46] and excluded three of them [44, 47, 48].

Included studies consisted of 2320 cases (1192 in progesterone group and 1128 in placebo-control group); SYNAPSE study and ProTECT-III respectively by Skolnick et al. and Wright et al. (in 2014) are the new phase 3, multi-centric, RCTs with the weight of 93.5% of whole cases [10, 11]. ProTECT-III halted in its secondary interim analysis, but SYNAPSE completed the predicted proposal and consists 51.5% of cases.

The analyses of favorable intervention outcome and mortality in these studies based on GOS report analysis in current method: favorably outcome (good recovery and moderate disability), mortality (vegetative state and death), the severe disability didn't included in the analysis. All of these studies analyzed their outcomes in a 6 month period but Wright et al. (in 2007), had a follow-up of 30 days [10, 11, 45, 46].

Intervention's side-effects also analyzed as the most happened for patients in each group as a whole but not on each of the side-effects solely. Also two studies didn't take part in this analysis. Skolnick et al.'s outcome results for adverse effects were different from case-control group's total number. It seems that five cases from control group have been analyzed in case group. An E-mail has been sent to the corresponding author for this confusing part, but till date, there is no reply [11]. Xiao et al. reported no adverse effects for the intervention [46].

The analyses showed no significant differences between progesterone and placebo groups in favorable treatment [(p = 0.75; RR 1.02, 95% CI 0.88–1.19; participants = 2320; studies = 4; I^2 = 53%) **Figure 2**], neither in mortalities [(p = 0.21; RR 0.77, 95% CI 0.50–1.17; participants = 2320; studies = 4; I^2 = 82%) **Figure 3**], nor in adverse effects analysis [(p = 085; RR 1.03, 95% CI 0.72–1.48; participants = 982; studies = 2; I^2 = 87%) **Figure 4**].

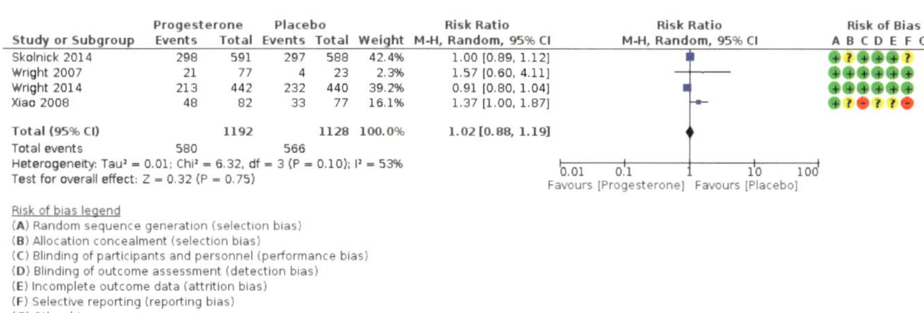

Figure 2.
Progesterone favorable outcome.

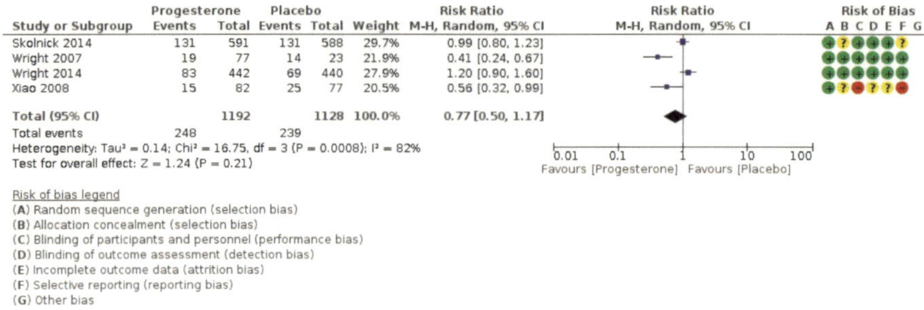

Figure 3.
Progesterone mortality.

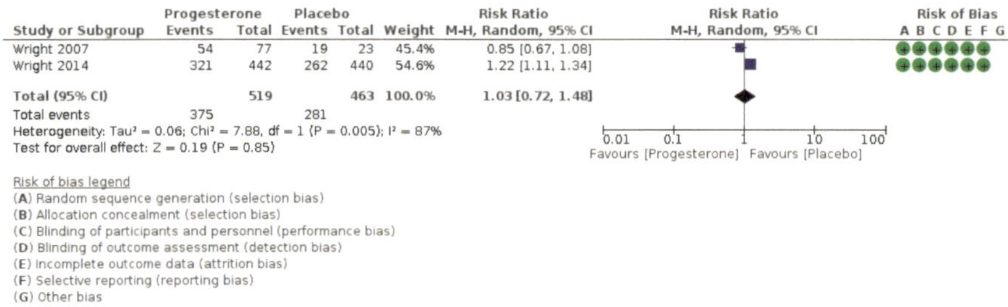

Figure 4.
Progesterone adverse-effects.

4.2.4 Monoaminergic agents

The Cochrane review of “Monoaminergic agonists for acute traumatic brain injury,” first established in 2006, and updated later on, till its last update was in 2011 didn't included any studies [19]. Search results didn’t collect any new studies.

4.2.5 Erythropoietin (EPO)

The primary search results for this topic, consists of a review on in-vitro and in-vivo studies till 2009 [49]. One retrospective case-control study [50] and four prospective RCTs [20, 22, 51, 52]; two of these studies were reports of a same phase-III multi-centric placebo-control trial known as EPO-TBI, and Nichol et al.’s reporting was more complete than the other one, which persuades authors to exclude Presneil et al. from quantitative analysis [21, 22]. Abrishamkar et al.’s paper has been excluded from meta-analysis too, due to its restricted study design on male patients [20].

The whole studies population analysis related to Aloizos et al. and Nichol et al. were 645 patients [21, 51]. Both studies followed patient up to 6 months analyzing total better outcomes of patients showed no significant difference between study groups [(p = 0.30; MD 1.22, 95% CI −1.09–3.53; participants = 638; studies = 2; I^2 = 99%) **Figure 5**], also EPO-TBI trial’s GOS reporting outcome showed no significant difference too [(p = 0.90; RR 1.01, 95% CI 0.87–1.17; participants = 596; studies = 1; I^2 = 0%) **Figure 6**]. Mortality and vegetative-state analysis, was significantly skewed toward intervention group [(p = 0.04; RR 0.65, 95% CI 0.43–0.98; participants = 644; studies = 2; I^2 = 0%) **Figure 7**]; while side-effect analysis showed nearly significant less vascular side effects in intervention group [(p = 0.06; RR 0.86, 95% CI 0.73–1.00; participants = 603; studies = 1; I^2 = 100%) **Figure 8**] and no significant difference in non-vascular side-effects between two groups of EPO-TBI

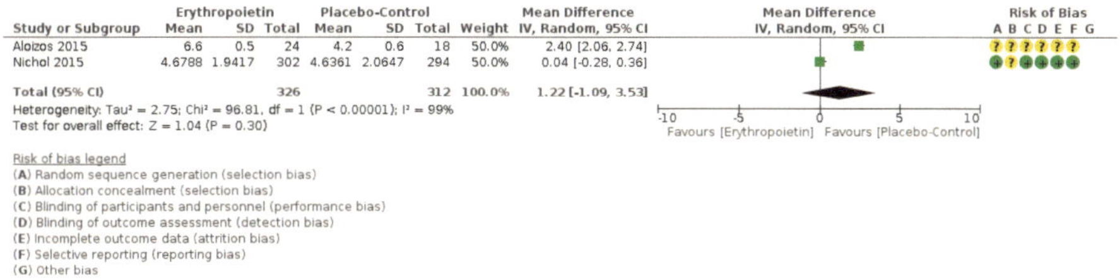

Figure 5.
Erythropoietin total outcome assessment.

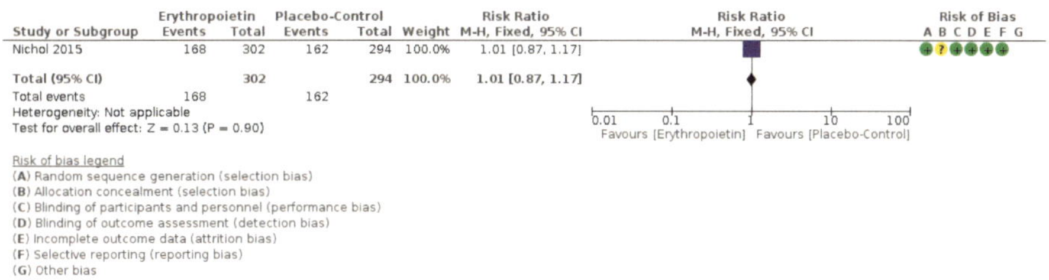

Figure 6.
Erythropoietin favorable outcome.

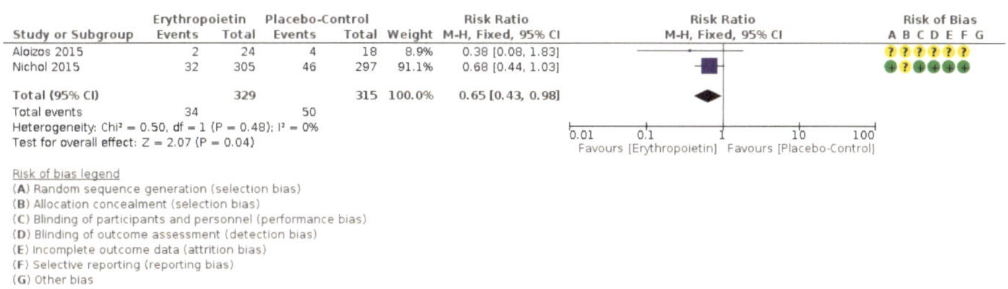

Figure 7.
Erythropoietin mortality.

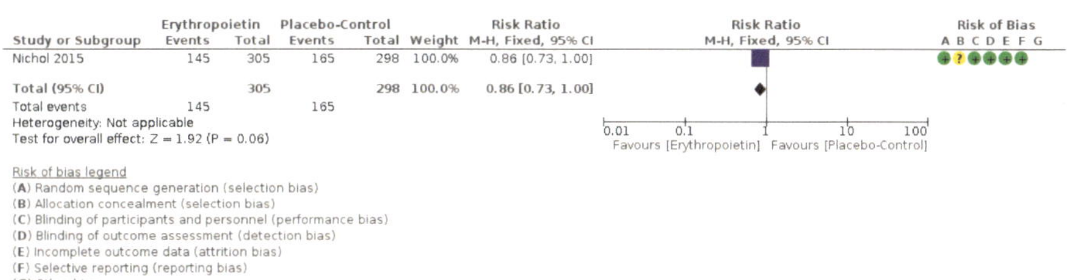

Figure 8.
Erythropoietin vascular side-effects.

trial [(p = 0.73; RR 0.93, 95% CI 0.62–1.39; participants = 603; studies = 1; I^2 = 0%) **Figure 9**], there was no side effect report in Aloizos et al. [51].

4.2.6 Magnesium sulfate and other magnesium salts

An updated review on magnesium, published in 2009 [23]; and no new studies been established in current review's search results after that timeline, the only study which was not mentioned in Vink et al. paper, was a pilot study on pediatric population with severe TBI, to maintain magnesium's feasibility and bio-availably for this population [52]. The common result of these studies, could be summarized

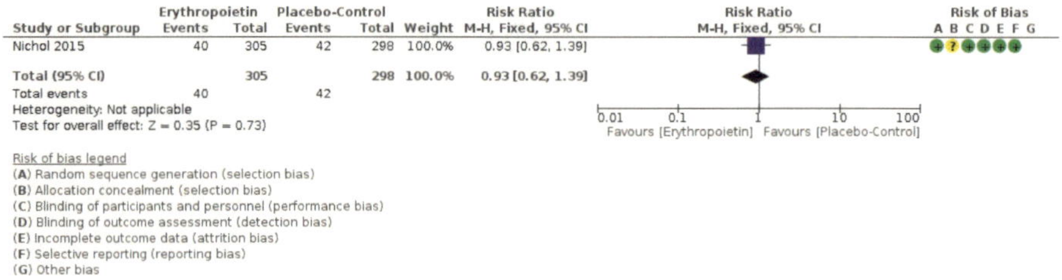

Figure 9.
Erythropoietin non-vascular side-effects.

as despite pre-clinical in-vivo studies of magnesium concentration in cerebrospinal fluid (CSF), that decline after acute TBI, and magnesium administration enhances its disposition in this field; no BBB feasibility seen in human studies for magnesium, and predicted mechanisms of actions for this intervention on human-beings are out of clinical evidence support [23, 52].

4.2.7 Cerebrolysin

There was a cohort-study by Wong et al. and a phase-II RCT by Chen et al. for cerebrolysin use in the search results [24, 53], also an ongoing huge multi-centric study held from third quarter of 2015 as well [54]. Cohort study, followed 42 patients with moderate to severe TBI, in 1:1 ratio, and report the outcomes in GOS scale after 6 months, which resulted in 67% good outcomes with cerebrolysin: placebo ratio of 19:14 in both study groups. The RCT reported cognitive outcomes with Mini-Mental Status Examination (MMSE) and Cognitive Abilities Screening Instrument (CASI) scales for mild TBI patients after 3 months that showed significant favorable outcome in intervention group [($p = 0.02$; MD −13.40, 95% CI −24.87 to −1.93; participants = 32; studies = 1; $I^2 = 0\%$) **Figure 10**].

4.2.8 Citicoline (CDP-choline) and other cholinergics

Articles related to citicoline intervention published from 1991–2014 [55–58]. Zafonte et al.'s study was a huge multicentric study a.k.a. COBRIT (citicoline brain injury treatment) and halted in its forth interim analysis due to non-significant outcome differences between placebo and intervention groups, but patients followed up to 180 days after injury, that 180 day's results are included in this review's analysis. Maldonado et al. and Shokouhi et al. studies didn't have placebo group, they were case-control studies, both included patients with severe or moderate acute TBI (216 and 58 patients respectively) [56, 57]. Leon-Carrion et al. study was a limited RCT of 10 patients for assessing neurocognitive effects of citicoline [55]. COBRIT planned to enroll 1292 patients, which halted in its forth interim analysis with 1213 patients randomized in two placebo and citicoline groups, the

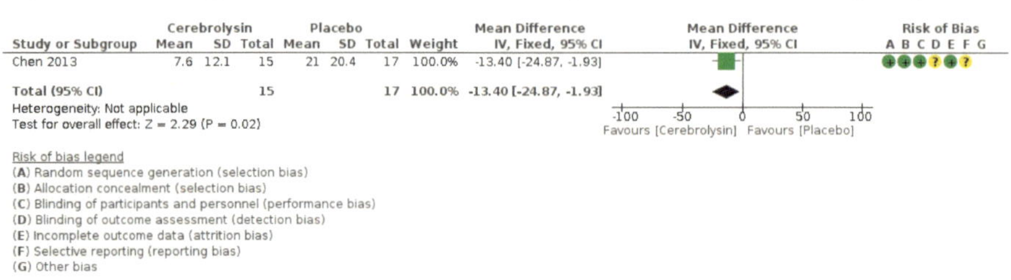

Figure 10.
Cognitive changes for cerebrolysin.

primary outcome assessment on day 90 of patients, was available for 996 cases, while 180-day outcome enrolled 902 cases [58].

In total, this meta-analysis included four studies with 1196 patients, which COBRIT study weighs about 75% of the analysis. The starting citicoline dose in studies was 2 g/day in Zafonte et al. and Shokouhi et al.'s trials, 1 g/day in Leon-Carrion et al.'s study, and 4 g/day in Maldonado et al.'s (that reduced to 3 g/day after day 3–4 of intervention and 2 g/day in case phlebitis would recognized).

Meta-analysis of outcomes showed no significant change in GOS outcome [(p = 0.76; RR 1.03, 95% CI 0.86–1.24; participants = 1128; studies = 2; I^2 = 71%) **Figure 11**], but significant favorable of neurocognitive changes in placebo-control group despite studies heterogeneity [($p < 0.00001$; SMD 1.00, 95% CI 0.75–1.25; participants = 971; studies = 3) **Figure 12**]. However the comparison of COBRIT study's days-90 and 180 GOS outcomes, demonstrated improvements in day 180 outcomes [58]. Mortality and vegetative-state outcomes were analyzed together in studies, which only two studies (Maldonado et al. and Zafonte et al.) reported these outcomes with no significant difference [(p = 0.96; RR 0.98, 95% CI 0.51–1.86; participants = 1429; studies = 2; I^2 = 67%) **Figure 13**]. The side-effects of intervention at all has no significant difference between trial groups either [(p = 0.53; RR 1.03, 95% CI 0.94–1.12; participants = 1429; studies = 2; I^2 = 57%) **Figure 14**].

4.2.9 NeuroAid

There was no trial for NeuroAid use in TBI.

4.2.10 Cyclosporine A (CysA)

Search strategies results, brought five articles for this topic; and all were prospective clinical trials, Brophy et al., Empey et al., and Mazzeo et al. (in 2008) reported and analyzed Cyclosporine's concentration and safety dose for human use

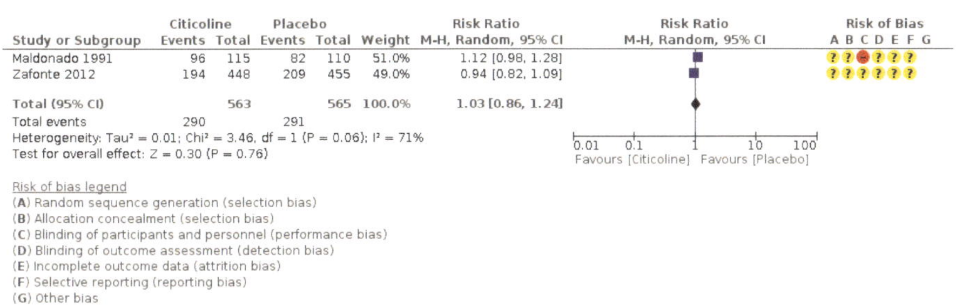

Figure 11.
Citicoline favorable outcome (GOS results).

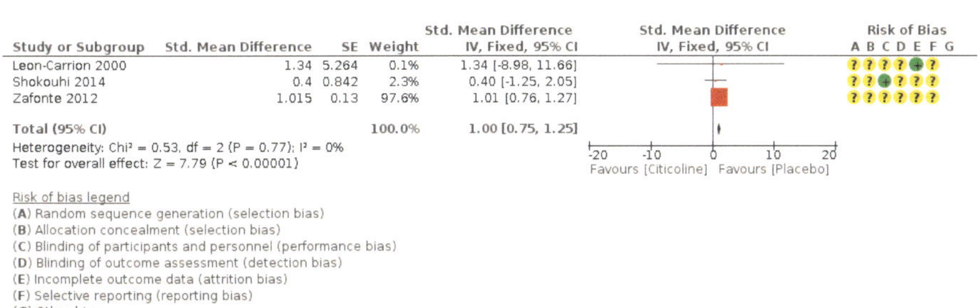

Figure 12.
Citicoline favorable outcome (at all).

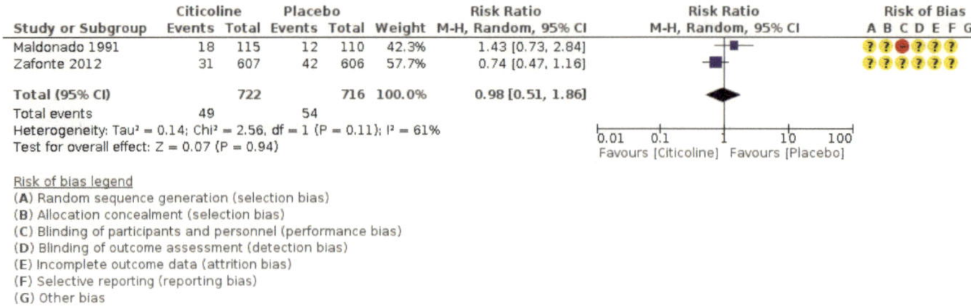

Figure 13.
Citicoline mortality.

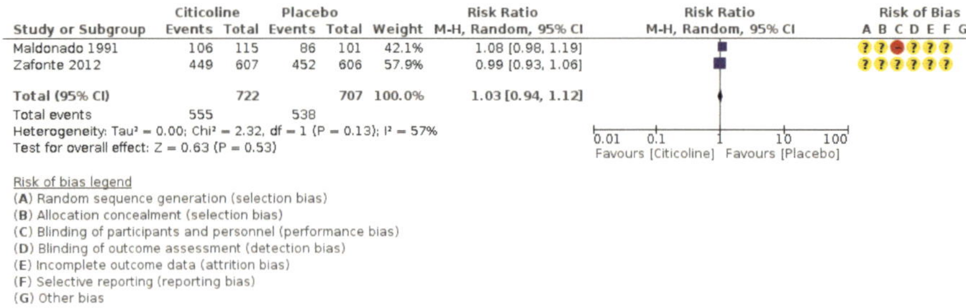

Figure 14.
Citicoline side-effects.

were [28, 59, 60]. The other two papers' population been analyzed at all were 89 patients [29, 61]. Cyclosporine's favorable GOS outcome analysis showed no significant difference between two interventional and placebo groups [(p = 0.83; RR 1.28, 95% CI 0.14–11.86; participants = 75; studies = 2; I^2 = 65%) **Figure 15**]; either there was no significant difference in mortalities [(p = 0.76; RR 1.17, 95% CI 0.443.12; participants = 89; studies = 2; I^2 = 0%) **Figure 16**] but CysA had significant effect on ICP control, and less ICP rise in comparison to placebo [(p = 0.01; RR 0.70, 95% CI 0.53–0.92; participants = 89; studies = 2; I^2 = 39%) **Figure 17**].

4.2.11 Rivastigmine

Three articles were related to this intervention in search results [30, 31, 62]. Silver et al. [31] was the continuation follow-up of Silver et al. [30] trial, which all placebo and rivastigmine group of 2006 study, got through rivastigmine intervention for 26 extra weeks, the results of this article, didn't differ significantly from the last report, so the 2009 study was excluded from the analysis; Tenovuo's study was

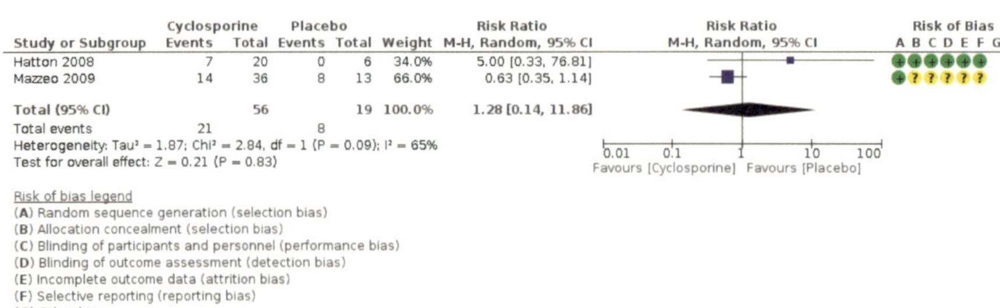

Figure 15.
Cyclosporine favorable outcome.

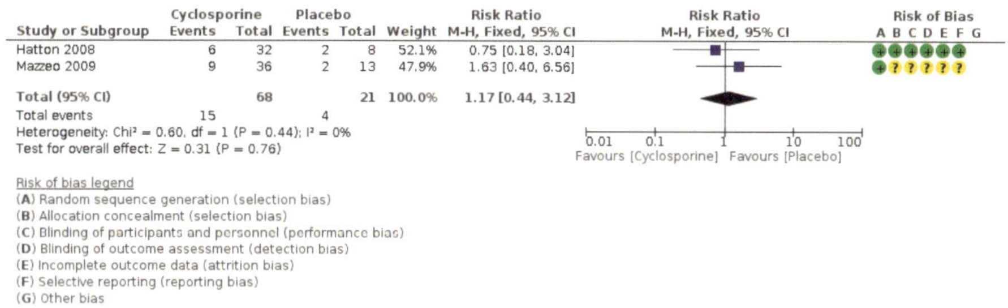

Figure 16.
Cyclosporine mortality.

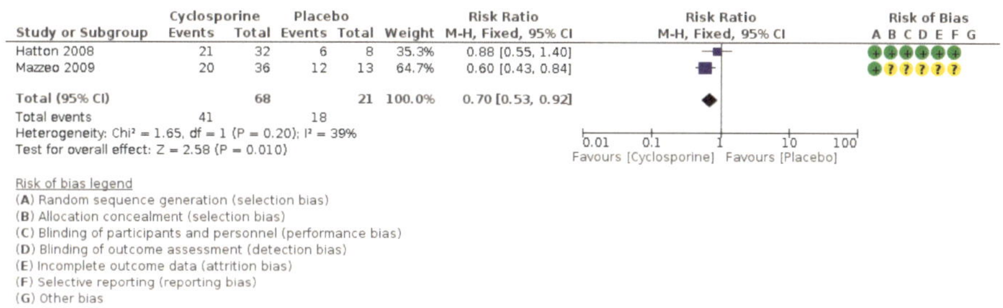

Figure 17.
Cyclosporine side effects (ICP rise).

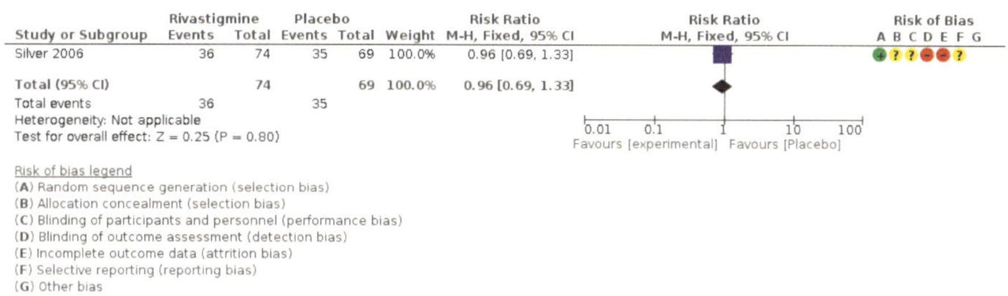

Figure 18.
Rivastigmine favorable outcome.

an out-patient clinic practice on 111 patients with three ChE-inh (Rivastigmine, Galantamine, and Donepezil), randomly assigned to patients by author, was excluded because of no placebo group, no blinding allocation statement and no obvious concealment reporting. Which all of these three articles lead results reporting to Silver et al. [30] trial, with 157 randomized patients in 77 placebo and 80 rivastigmine groups.

Silver et al. [30] study, has no mortality report in cases, but patients whom completed 12 weeks of trial time-line, were 70 in rivastigmine and 64 in placebo groups, also three patients in total lost to follow up (one in rivastigmine and two in placebo group); There was no significant difference for favorable outcome results of this intervention in comparison to placebo [(p = 0.80; RR 0.96, 95% CI 0.69–1.33; participants = 143; studies = 1; I^2 = 0%) **Figure 18**]. But authors stated that rivastigmine was efficient for more severe impaired patients in both 2006 and 2009 reports [30, 31]; it was analyzed as a sub-group analysis of 25% of patients and its raw results were not declared in the studies. Side-effect analysis show no meaningful difference too [(p = 0.74; RR 1.04, 95% CI 0.84–1.27; participants = 157; studies = 1; I^2 = 0%) **Figure 19**].

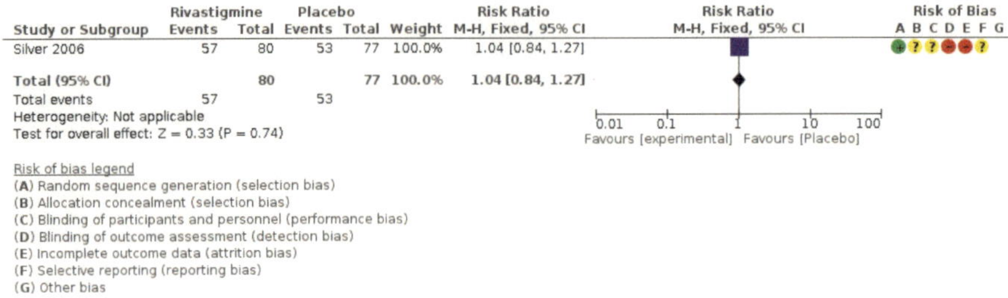

Figure 19.
Rivastigmine side effects.

4.2.12 Piracetam

Search results brought following three titles for this intervention "Clinical Evaluation of Nootropil (Piracetam) in Severe Craniocerebral Injuries," "Clinical trial of piracetam in disorders of consciousness due to head injury," and "A controlled clinical study piracetam V. Placebo in disorders of consciousness due to head injuries" but there was no achievement to their full-texts. However attempts to contact authors had no success too.

4.2.13 Miscellaneous findings

There were review-like studies and RCTs, further than these 12 categorized neuroprotectives, for TBI management, that a quick review of them proceeds in the following paragraphs

a. A 2013 "meta-analysis of treating acute traumatic brain injury with calcium channel blockers," of nine RCTs, showed slightly better outcome of placebo group, but it was not statistically significant ($p = 0.52$; RR 1.18, 95% CI 0.72–1.95; participants = 171; studies = 2; I2 = 52%), however there was no significant difference between intervention and placebo groups in mortalities ($p = 0.44$; RR 0.93, 95% CI 0.77–1.12; participants = 1337; studies = 5; I2 = 0%), nor adverse effects ($p = 0.33$; RR 1.11, 95% CI 0.90–1.37; participants = 1358; studies = 4; I2 = 0%) [63]. The former hypothesis of "The role of mitochondrial calcium uni-porter in neuroprotection in traumatic brain injury" may be disclaimed as a result of this meta-analysis [64].

b. A parallel study to COBRIT "Early trajectory of Psychiatric Symptoms after Traumatic Brain Injury: Relationship to patient and Injury Characteristic," show overall an improvement process of psychiatric characteristic of TBI patient over 180 days assessment, with better outcomes on days 30–90; better outcomes of female participants in comparison to males; not statistical significant but Hispanic's most and African-American's least improvement process in comparison to whites as the ethnic/race analysis' reference group [65].

   - Better significant emotion recognition training outcome by the mean of 11 years after TBI in facial affect recognition better than participants of stories group in comparison to control group, showed impaired cognitive abilities improvement in moderate to severe TBI patients in "A randomized controlled trial of emotion recognition training after traumatic brain injury" [66]; however hypothetical testing of stories group to assess their ability to infer and label their feelings in given scenarios, showed significant improvements. Patients responses to these emotional recognitions, was not favorable, as authors recommend further studies to instruct participants on how to response too [66].

- Hyperthermia after acute TBI, significantly results in unfavorable outcomes and mortality rates of especially severe head injured patients [67]; a Cochrane review of "Cooling for cerebral protection during brain surgery" didn't show significant result for this intervention [68], which might be due to different purposes of studies.

- And Finally a before-after clinical trial of 35 patients for "Effect of light music on physiological parameters of patients with traumatic brain injuries at intensive care units" using Dr. ArndStein's 70–80 metronome rhythmic melody, showed better significant physiologic outcomes in decreasing systolic and diastolic blood pressure, pulse rate, respiratory rate, arterial blood pressure and body temperature and increasing arterial oxygen saturation (<0.001); however pulse pressure decreasing was not significant [69].

4.2.14 Risk of bias in included studies

As a whole, "randomization part" of studies has a good assessment overall; however "allocation concealment" or "how blinding participants or personnel take place" didn't seem to be well reported. Finally RCTs reporting didn't accommodate well enough to CONSORT statement (i.e., this review study's tool for analyzing study reports). **Figures 20** and **21** are at a glance quick look assessment of risk of bias in included studies.

4.2.15 Effects of interventions

Overall, by the analysis of only phase-III studies results, no significant difference seen between neuroprotectives and placebo groups in favorable outcomes [(p = 0.30; RR 0.97, 95% CI 0.90–1.03; participants = 3560; studies = 4; I^2 = 0%) **Figure 22**]; or mortalities [(p = 0.51; RR 0.92, 95% CI 0.73–1.17; participants = 3876; studies = 4; I^2 = 52%) **Figure 23**].

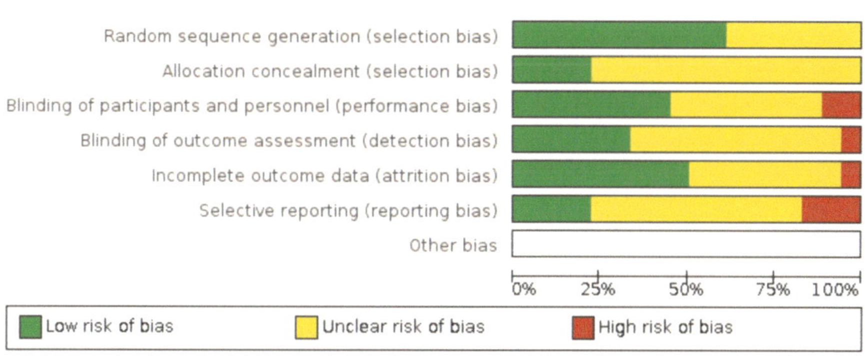

Figure 20.
Risk of biases graph: review author's judgments about each risk of bias item presented as percentages across all included studies.

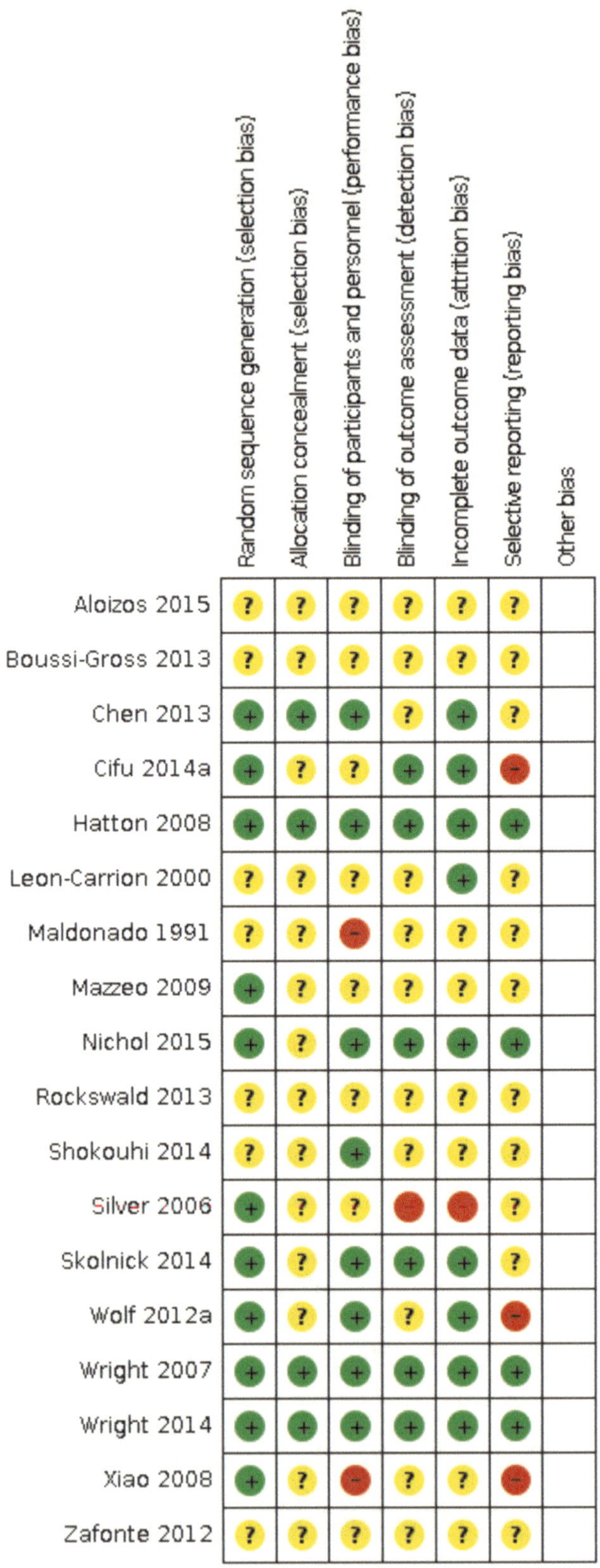

Figure 21.
Risk of biases summary: review author's judgments about each risk of bias item for each included study.

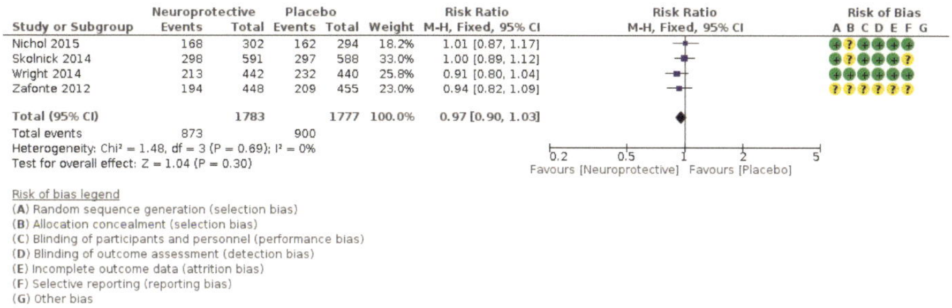

Figure 22.
Phase-III neuroprotectives favorable outcome.

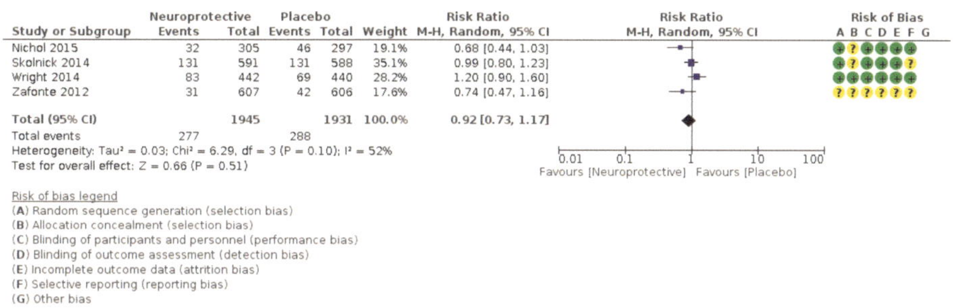

Figure 23.
Phase-III neuroprotectives mortality (CRASH 2005 not included).

5. Discussion

5.1 Summary of main results

5.1.1 Oxygen

Despite other trials of oxygen intervention in acute phase TBI, Rockswald et al. study's new design in combination of HBO_2/NBH, rather than solely attempt of each one results in better and significant outcomes [43]; it could be a new recommendation for future trials of acute phase TBI management, as its mortality report was the same as past trials, but with better GOS outcome [1, 43].

Boussi-Gross et al. study's improvement results in cognitive function of mild chronic TBI patients despite other DoD-/VA-related studies' results may be due to differences in civilian and service member populations of each study design, probable posttraumatic syndrome disorder (PTSD) symptoms of DoD/VA members, and different assessment tools; also, controversies of eye problem conditioning between Cifu et al. and Wolf et al. may resolve in a large group study with a common manifest of study objectives and participant evaluation [37, 38, 40–42].

In conclusion, there were lots of controversies between oxygen phase-II trials till now, but no multi-centric phase-III trial been conducted for this intervention, the one is strongly recommended also in a normal population and not just for DoD/VAs [41]. A Trial of HBO_2/NBH—(sham) control design may have most cost-beneficence than other kinds of solo intervention trials especially in acute phase TBI management [43]. Using oxygen (especially HBO_2) in chronic management of TBI has no enough evidences yet.

5.1.2 Corticosteroids

CRASH study's results that weigh about 95% of the Alderson's Cochrane review in "Corticosteroids for acute traumatic brain injury—last revised 2009," made the fact of increasing mortalities in TBI, by using corticosteroids [4]; no new trials found on steroids effect for TBI after these papers.

Current review's applicability on using corticosteroids for CNS acute traumas, leads to another Cochrane review of "Steroids for acute spinal cord injury—last revised 2012" [13]; however these conditions (TBI and SCI) may coincide (dual-diagnoses). So what are the practical recommendations for these situations?

According to Bracken's review "Methylprednisolone sodium succinate must be started within 8 hours of injury, using an initial bolus of 30 mg/kg by IV for 15 minutes followed 45 minutes later by a continuous infusion of 5.4 mg/kg/hour for 24 hours. Further improvement in motor function recovery has been shown to occur when the maintenance therapy is extended for 48 hours. This is particularly evident when the initial bolus dose could only be administered 3–8 hours after injury"; dosage and limited time of intervention for SCI patients, mentioned in the review by contemplate of situations with cohesion of TBI and SCI literally 16–59% [70], therefore challenging decision making on using corticosteroids (especially Methylprednisolone, as recommended in the review) on these conditions needs awareness of reviews results combination. It's suggested to use the recommended methylprednisolone protocol for dual-diagnose patients only in the initial bolus dose timing of 3–8 hours after acute injury, following therapy for only 48 hours; neither other corticosteroids nor extensive use of this protocol, are not suggested or acceptable for dual-diagnose patients management, also Nott et al. study brings hopes in cognitive behavior of dual-diagnosed ones [70], that discussed by social effects of condition in the study, this may persuade health-care practitioner and cost-benefit analyst about using this intervention for dual-diagnoses.

5.1.3 Progesterone

SYNAPSE and ProTECT-III trials results for progesterone, changed the former vision of this intervention's effect on TBI management, as CRASH trial did for corticosteroid in 2005.

Progesterones are gonadal steroids, and assume to have been more favorable in neurodegenerative disorders like multiple sclerosis (MS), Alzheimer disease (AD), and maybe TBI, i.e., neurodegenerative effects of microglia after injury and induced inflammatory response in whole body [14, 16, 71], as mentioned by Beyer [15].

Leucht et al. and Burns et al. studies results are good challenging statements for current visions of pharmaceutical interventions for major chronic disorders and central nervous system (CNS) injuries respectively [9, 12]. The pharmaceutical interventions failure in huge phase-III trials for TBI in the last decade (i.e., from CRASH 2005 to EPO-TBI 2015), even as smoothly penetration of progesterone through BBB to take its promising effects in pre-clinical studies [10, 11, 14, 15, 17, 18], made this statement from Wright et al. who designed and proceed three trials of progesterone use in TBI [10, 45, 47] "Despite these design strategies and extensive efforts, the trial did not confirm the efficacy of progesterone in patients with acute TBI. It is possible that the heterogeneity of the injury, confounding preexisting conditions, and characteristics of individual patients (e.g., resilience), which can be well controlled in animal models, play too large a role to overcome in human disease. Approaches are needed to reduce heterogeneity, but they come at the cost of more homogeneous pathological findings and decreased generalization of the results. Success at translating from bench to bedside may require new paradigms, including innovative clinical-trial methods (e.g., adaptive designs and profiling of patients who have a response) in early-phase clinical trials to identify effective drug doses and timing (e.g., pre-hospital administration), the use of targeted outcomes based on the mechanism of injury, and rigorous preclinical multicentric trials in animals that better simulate subsequent human trials and make more accurate predictions regarding results." [10] "From Bench to Bed," "From Mice to Mind"; these statements declare incompatibility of basic studies with clinical trials; the basic science consortium approach, is one of good options for pharmaceutical intervention selection on human beings trials, it's on the way, as part of Combat Casualty Care Research Program-Operational Brain Trauma Therapy Consortium [11].

Concluding all these results together, may associate the future attempts on medicine to cellular-molecular field of bio-medicine in all of its era, as well as trauma management [9]. Review results should declare that using progesterone in the recommended I.V. doses has no significant beneficial effects than placebo; recommendation of using progesterone for pediatric patients in TBI insults [16], has no proof, as there is no structured RCT for that, and this age group's recovery of TBI effects, may naturally take place with controlling the damage by current guidelines. "Combination therapy of 17-Beta-E2 and Progesterone while applying a basis of Emulsion I.V. together with Omega-3 fatty acids, using high short-term dosages of treatments rather than normal long-term treatments" mentioned by Beyer as request of expertise-comment for his interests and experience since 1988 on Gonadal Steroids use for CNS problems [15] may present the clue for further researches in this field. Combination therapy of progesterone and vitamin D, especially in aged TBI patients [10, 14] is not proved in human cases, and beneficence of this combination recommended therapy, might be questioned for not significant efficacy of progesterone use in lately human phase-III RCTs; however another RCTs should hold for vitamin D use for TBI patients to verify this statement.

5.1.4 Monoaminergic agents

Cochrane review for this topic didn't include any articles, also there was no new studies in this review's search results too, and as they recommended in their article "in the absence of clear evidence of benefit from Neuroprotective drug use, there is an urgent need to explore other potential modulators of late outcome from TBI. The reported results of these studies require replication in larger studies, extended to other groups including more severely injured patients, and children" would be the clue of further researches and trials.

5.1.5 Erythropoietin (EPO)

The total analysis and results of this topic demonstrate that, it reduces mortality rates but no significant efficacy of EPO rather than placebo or control groups is noted; also EPO-TBI resulted in side-effects, which didn't report in other two trials [20, 21, 51], that might be due to EPO-TBI's higher EPO dose use (40,000 IU up to 3 doses) in comparison to 10,000 IU for 7 days of Aloizos et al. and 1000 IU in 6 doses during 2 weeks of Abrishamkar et al. There were side effects in placebo group of EPO-TBI trial too; that challenges this statement. Nearly significant better outcome of side-effects for EPO group in Nichol et al. EPO-TBI trial is far away from last expectations of EPO trials [21, 49] that confirms Leucht et al. statement on drugs complexity effect [12]. All three trials administered the intervention through subcutaneous (S.C.) route, as Abrishamkar et al. declared, despite LAB trials, it's nearly impossible to gather Intra-Ventricular route for agent administration in edematous TBI brain [20].

Final conclusion on this topic, otherwise its prospective phase-III multi-centric placebo-controlled RCT, cannot obviously be presented, due to different dose of interventions between studies (i.e., more than recommended does 1000–30,000 IU in EPO-TBI trial [21, 51]; better outcomes in mortality-rate and side-effects reduction for intervention group; But overall, it showed better outcome in placebo group, which makes the clinical decision-making a challenge on using EPO for acute TBI. It should be recommended to conduct another prospective phase-III multi-centric placebo-controlled RCT with intervention dose of no more than 30,000 IU during EPO-administration to conduct better decision about choosing this intervention wisely for acute TBI assaults.

5.1.6 Magnesium sulfate and other magnesium salts

Magnesium beneficence for human beings through its CSF concentration didn't proved with the former trials, and Vink et al. reported the fact in 2009 [23]. Further trials on magnesium concentration in CSF may conducted via its administration through Intra Ventricular route, to find out its probable Neuroprotective effect, however it seems not to be successful [20].

5.1.7 Cerebrolysin

Limited evidences for this intervention's effect on TBI patients, also in different severities of TBI, mild TBI in RCT study and moderate to severe TBI in cohort study [24, 55], couldn't investigate its reliability for generalized use recommendation in TBIs; Cerebrolysin Asian Pacific Trial in Acute Brain Injury and Neurorecovery (CAPTAIN) results [54] is going to lead the future responsibilities and decisions to use this intervention in TBI situations.

5.1.8 Citicoline (CDP-choline) and other cholinergics

COBRIT study for citicoline seems to be like CRASH, SYNAPSE and ProTECT-III or EPO-TBI, as it was a huge multicentric placebo-control RCT of citicoline, its halt in forth interim analysis, may resulted to less participant of patients in follow-up process, but it was none of significantly difference between groups' analysis, overall assessment of outcomes didn't demonstrate any significant effect of citicoline favorable especially in GOS, yet in COBRIT study's assessment of GOS for day-90 and 180, improvements are slightly better but not significant at all (from $p = 0.97$ to $p = 0.43$), there is significant improvement of placebo-control group patients in neurocognitive state rather than intervention group. Yet neither mortality nor side-effects of intervention versus control groups were significant.

Maldonado et al. study was the more notable one after Zafonte et al. COBRIT in these search results; this study, Leon-Carrion et al. and Shokouhi et al. studies' beneficence in citicoline use for severe and moderate TBIs, questioned by COBRIT overall outcomes both in day-90 and 180 outcomes [55–58]. Also a significant better outcome change was obvious in mildly complicated cases on day-180 outcome in COBRIT study [58]. Heterogeneity of intervention doses and outcome assessments in included studies surrounded by Zafonte et al. Study's results; though current use of citicoline for TBI in acute or chronic phase, is no more recommended by the results of this review, however it may have neurocognitive beneficiaries for mild TBI, that decision of using this experiment on these conditions, belongs to attending physician's opinion and other assessments.

5.1.9 NeuroAid

Trials on Neuroaid for brain injury conditions mostly studied its effects on stroke brain injuries; none of current study's search results, related to Neuroaid use in TBI; that may suggest the clue for future trials.

5.1.10 Cyclosporine A (CysA)

Cyclosporine A's use may prevent ICP rise or reduce it, in comparison to placebo as this analysis showed. However there is no significant effect of its use in 6-month favorable outcomes or mortality rates. Also cohort study groups of Hatton et al. and other drug concentration studies confirm that best blood and cerebrospinal fluid (CSF) CysA depositions resulted from its high doses and fortunately the wide therapeutic window [28, 59–61]. Both of the included studies have a 5 mg/kg intervention on their design protocols, also Hatton et al. recommended a 2.5 mg/kg bolus dose in 2 hours of TBI insult following by 5 mg/kg/day for 72 hours, as optimal dosing strategy for further clinical trials study design. As there would be a huge multi-centric, prospective, phase-III RCT for CysA after National Institute of Health (NIH) proves its proposal [29]; that might bring future evidences on using this intervention for TBI (especially acute) management.

5.1.11 Rivastigmine

Rivastigmine and other ChE-inh use for TBI, mostly known for their cognitive behavioral effects, and their trials take part in chronic TBI managements, Tenovuo's study didn't show a significant difference between three drugs that patients assigned to use, but mostly preferred Galantamine for its fewer side effects [62]. Silver et al. (both 2006 and 2009 studies) with 157 patients and better study design in comparison to Tenovuo's, didn't show significant difference of rivastigmine and placebo groups at all, but in severe impaired patients. These results support the need of more RCTs especially multi-centric phase-III RCTs of rivastigmine and other ChE-inh for chronic TBI management in severe impaired patients, the recommended protocol as Silver et al. Stated, is to start with 3 mg of rivastigmine/day and slowly increase to maximum dose of 12 mg/day if the previous dose was well tolerated for at least 4 weeks. Routine use of rivastigmine for chronic TBI management is not recommended, as it has no significant effect for patients rather than placebo, as current evidences declared.

5.1.12 Piracetam

There were studies for this intervention but no achievement to their full-texts, it may be one of this review's reporting biases, which no clinical judgment may presented for this intervention.

5.1.13 Miscellaneous findings

Following statements are recommendations for "Miscellaneous Findings" section of "Results" section of the study:

- Improvement in psychiatric assessments of TBI patient, after assault differ between individuals, there should be supportive psychological first aid (PFA) tools for primary survivors of the assault; a Johns Hopkins University's course of PFA-RAPID which stands for Rapport and Reflective Listening, Assessment of Needs, Prioritization, Intervention, Disposition; is available at https://www.coursera.org/course/psychfirstaid to triage and primary effective intervene of health-care providers for trauma assaults survivors, as further than the insult, sub-acute complications during recovery of patients, especially in two-third of severe impaired TBI patients [72], may have affects on their family's life too.

- Cerebral and body cooling for acute TBI impaired patients, may have better outcomes in patients survival and reducing mortality rates, due to significant unfavorable outcomes and mortality rates of high fevered patients after acute TBI in Li et al. study; a strong evidence of phase-III multi-centric international RCT, needed to prove this statement.

- Music-therapy use for TBI patient, seem to have better outcomes in physiologic parameters, however other double-blinded RCTs need to prove this statement. However Maleki et al. study's aim was not to assess participants outcomes; as well actual efficacy of this intervention on patients outcomes, might took under survey too [9, 73, 74].

5.2 Overall completeness and applicability of evidence

All of RCTs checked with CONSORT 2010 checklist; the applicability of this tool for further analysis of probable biases from participant randomization to outcome report used on each of the included studies as well.

5.3 Potential biases in the review process

Primary database search strategy, didn't consist interventions as search keywords separately, the consultation with a medical librarian, persuade authors to revise the strategy with search of Piracetam, NeuroAid and Citicoline (as commonly used Neuroprotectives in their tertiary center, and for meta-analysis purpose of these interventions), the re-run search strategy added few (about 7–10) records in each database search, that skim review on their title and abstracts (duplicated records, assessed with Zotero reference manager software for exclusion), didn't show significant change of eligible studies, and further search on all interventions as solo keywords, didn't take place. Current meta-analyses based on second search strategy results. This may be a selection bias of this study and future reviews should be aware of this bias; another probable bias in this review was in reporting outcomes and mortalities analyses; Authors decide to report GOS or GOS-E outcomes analyses in two groups: (1) favorable outcome, which consists of good outcome and mild disability (GOS 4,5 and GOS-E 5-8) outcome; and (2) mortalities, that reported vegetative state and mortalities analysis (GOS 1,2 and GOS-E 1,2). Some of the articles, reported severe disability, vegetative-state and mortality outcomes together; if it was possible to get special reports on outcomes, analyses get through them, but if not, they'd been analyzed as the original article's authors decision.

5.4 Agreements and disagreements with other studies or reviews

This review was a brand-new in interventions analyses for TBI (mostly acute) management; other previous reviews based on significant intervention's effect analysis; some parts of this review used the former reviews or meta-analyses results conducting new one, are referred through the text.

5.5 Final pluralization

Overall conclusion of these results and outcome findings of neuroprotective agents for traumatic brain injury management could be summarized as follows:

a. Oxygen using for acute management of TBI to reduce mortality rates is obvious, however no significant change seen in favorable outcomes, if a setting has HBO_2 resource available, combined use of HBO_2/NBH, may have better patient outcomes than using HBO_2 or NBH solely; recommended approach for this facility is "combined HBO2/NBH treatment, which consisted of 100% FiO_2 delivered for 60 minutes at 1.5 ATA followed by 3 hours at 1.0 ATA" [43]; also there is no significant evidence for using HBO_2 in chronic TBI management.

b. Corticosteroid use in solo acute TBI management is prohibited, as its increased risk of mortalities; in dual-diagnosed patients (TBI and SCI together), corticosteroid use, should be obtained by this protocol [13]:

    i. patient came through 2–3 hours after assault (if longer, should not be obtained)

    ii. only methylprednisolone (other corticosteroids, has no beneficent effect in SCI management) with following protocol should be administered through IV route:

        - Bolus dose: 30 mg/kg in 15 minutes,

        - Following drip of: 5.4 mg/kg/day for the next 24–48 hours.

c. Current routine use of citicoline in acute TBI is no more supported, while no significant difference in comparison to placebo been reported. Citicoline use for managing neurocognitive conditions of chronic TBI, depends on attended physician's evaluation of patient's condition and local setting's evidence based medicine (EBM) community's decision. Rather its probable benefice in mild TBI patients, it's not recommended for all severity of TBI, while significant improvements seen in placebo group.

d. Using of Cyclosporine A for ICP control, depends on the setting's available resources, and attending physician's point of view, there is no other significant difference for its favorable outcome in comparison to placebo. it should be recommend to administer through IV route by following protocol in acute TBI management [61]:

    i. Bolus dose: 2.5 mg/kg in 2 hours,

    ii. Following drip of: 5 mg/kg/day for the next 72 hours.

e. Rivastigmine use for chronic TBI management of neurocognitive conditions, had some beneficence in severe impaired participants through phase-II trials of 3 mg/day and slowly increasing to 12 mg/day by adding 1.5 mg/day to previous dose if tolerated for 4 weeks of last dose [30].

f. Other neuroprotective agents use for acute or chronic management of TBI, has no field of support yet.

6. Conclusions

6.1 Recommendations for practice

To use oxygen in acute management of TBI in order to reduce mortality rates seems to be obvious, however no significant change seen in favorable outcomes; corticosteroid use in solo acute TBI management is prohibited, as it increases risk of mortalities, however in dual-diagnosed patients (TBI & SCI together), corticosteroid use, should be obtained by a protocol introduced by Bracken et al. Current routine use of citicoline in acute TBI is no more supported, while no significant difference in comparison to placebo been reported. Cyclosporine A usage for ICP control, depends on the available resources, and attending physician's point of view; Rivastigmine use for chronic TBI management of neurocognitive conditions, had some beneficence in severe impaired participants. However other Neuroprotective agents use for acute or chronic management of TBI, has no field of support yet and they needed more researches and trials.

6.2 Recommendations for research

Lastly phase-III RCTs for TBI management, change the former evidences of Neuroprotective agents use (i.e., CRASH 2005 for corticosteroid [4], COBRIT 2012 for citicoline [58]. SYNAPSE 2014 [11] and ProTECT 2014 [10] for Progesterone and EPO-TBI 2015 for erythropoietin [21]; despite current process of phase-I to phase-III (IV) new drug evaluation to use in human-beings, it should be recommended to skip phase-II trials for TBI related studies; heterogeneity of the condition, make its accurate interpretation so difficult in restricted single-centered phase-II trials. Scheduling large double (or more)-blinded huge multi-centric international phase-III RCTs, including low-income countries too as recommended by Menon in "Unique challenges in clinical trials in traumatic brain injury" [75], with acceptable design of interim analyses for number needed to harm (NNH) and number needed to treat (NNT) at regular checkpoints, seem to have more accuracy and cost-beneficent effects than current known processes. There was no strong-evidenced well-designed trials for these interventions:

- Combined therapy of HBO_2/NBH
- Monoaminergics;
- "High-dose, short-time administration of progesterone with 17-Beta-E2 in emulsion of Omega-3," as an expert advice for future studies [15] rather than SYNAPSE and ProTECT results;
- Administering magnesium solutions via Intra-Ventricular or other achievable routes in TBI patients for rising its concentration in TBI patient's CSF;
- Rivastigmine use for chronic management of severe impaired neurocognitive conditions;
- Cerebral or body cooling, especially in severely impaired patients of acute TBI assault.

Also a Cerebrolysin phase-III trial is in the ongoing-list of current study [54]. And despite NeuroAid's trials for stroke injured brain, there was no trial (even phase-II) of this intervention for TBI.

Cellular-molecular experiences in CNS conditions, has not been provided acceptable outcomes for TBI to date, but as a recommendation of an expert "there is potential for TBI" as "mirror pathophysiology of some of the other conditions," despite "the lack of sensitive outcome measures" there is hope to "promote at least some improvement in recovery of function via immunomodulation and promoting plasticity" [9].

It's also recommended for RCT authors to use CONSORT-assessment guidelines in their study designs and paper reports; and report clinical outcomes of mild, moderate and severe suffered acute TBI patients in separate subgroup analyses, which an eight-pointed GOS-E reporting scale is preferred to five-pointed GOS one [75]; till better outcome assessment tool been developed; however studies on hypotheses of drugs concentration in serum, or assessing physiological parameters of patients; resulted in no more significant outcome of TBI patients in large phase-III studies.

Acknowledgements

Our kind regards and appreciations belong to Mrs. Fathifar and Mr. Saeidi, the librarians of Tabriz Nutritional Sciences Faculty and Tabriz University of Medical Sciences Central Library, who also commented to our primary search strategy to revise it into better applicability and help us come through the full-texts of related articles; also Mr. Ahadi, MA in English literature and language, who reviewed our primary draft and his precious recommendations made better outfit of this manuscript. The following authors, make the meaningfulness of "Standing on the shoulders of Giants" & "Open Accessed World Wide Web (WWW)" for us; by providing their own papers' full-texts for our study, despite the limitations of known routes in WWW, via www.researchgate.net; our appreciations belongs to them and to whom else endeavors on making these Ottos possible: Dr. David B. Arciniegas, Dr. Lisa Anne Brenner, Dr. Jose Leon-Carion, Dr. Andrew I.R. Maas & Dr. Olli Tenovuo. Prof. Cordian Beyer's Comments on "Gonadal Esteroids and Progesterone" as his most experience on the topic since 1988, may bring new hopes in this era; Dr. Burns' comments on probable effectiveness of Cellular Medicine for TBI management, should be valuable route of future studies & researches. And We used bunch of Libre/Open Source Software to surf the web, collect information, analyze data & publish the paper; our kind pleasures belongs to alumni of "Mozilla FireFox," "LibreOffice," "Zotero," "uGet" & "Cochrane RevMan" (hope the last one some day would be published under software freedoms Two and Three too); and "Richard Stallman" founder of "Free Software Foundation (www.fsf.org)," for bringing these useful elaborate software and the philosophy of software freedom for human beings. Also Our Kind regards and appreciations belong to Ms. Rozmari Marijan for her really kind and supportive help, feed-backs and follow-ups for performing this manuscript of Intech-Open format, and made the meaningfulness of "Publishing Science in Peace."

Conflict of interest

This chapter is the reporting result of a GP graduation thesis from Tabriz University of Medical Sciences, which was defended on June 2016 under thesis number 92/1-1/6.

Author details

Mohammad Meshkini[1,2]*, Ali Meshkini[1,3] and Homayoun Sadeghi-Bazargani[1,4]

1 Road Traffic Injury Research Center, Tabriz University of Medical Sciences, Tabriz, Iran

2 Emergency Medicine Resident, Emergency Medicine Department, Iran University of Medical Sciences, Tehran, Iran

3 Department of Neurological-Surgery, Faculty of Medicine, Imam-Reza Hospital, Tabriz University of Medical Sciences, Tabriz, Iran

4 Department of Bio-statistics and Epidemiology, Faculty of Health and Nutrition Sciences, Tabriz University of Medical Sciences, Tabriz, Iran

*Address all correspondence to: meshkini522@gmail.com

References

[1] Bennett MH, Trytko B, Jonker B. Hyperbaric oxygen therapy for the adjunctive treatment of traumatic brain injury. Cochrane Database of Systematic Reviews. 2012. [Internet]. [cited 2015 Dec 27];12. Available from: http://dev.biologists.org/content/3/4/326.short

[2] Roberts I, Schierhout G. Hyperventilation therapy for acute traumatic brain injury. In: The Cochrane Collaboration, editor. Cochrane Database of Systematic Reviews. Chichester, UK: John Wiley & Sons, Ltd; 1997. [Internet]. [cited 2015 Dec 26]. Available from: http://doi.wiley.com/10.1002/14651858.CD000566

[3] Thompson K, Pohlmann-Eden B, Campbell Leslie A, Abel H. Pharmacological treatments for preventing epilepsy following traumatic head injury (Review). Cochrane Database of Systematic Reviews. 2015. [Internet]. [cited 2015 Dec 26];8. Available from: http://journals.lww.com/ccmjournal/Abstract/2010/05000/Long_term_mortality_and_quality_of_life_in_sepsis_.6.aspx

[4] Alderson P, Roberts I. Corticosteroids for acute traumatic brain injury. In: The Cochrane Collaboration, editor. Cochrane Database of Systematic Reviews. Chichester, UK: John Wiley & Sons, Ltd; 2005. [Internet]. [cited 2015 Dec 26]. Available from: http://doi.wiley.com/10.1002/14651858.CD000196.pub2

[5] Ma J, Huang S, Qin S, You C. Progesterone for acute traumatic brain injury. In: The Cochrane Collaboration, editor. Cochrane Database of Systematic Reviews. Chichester, UK: John Wiley & Sons, Ltd; 2012. [Internet]. [cited 2015 Dec 26]. Available from: http://doi.wiley.com/10.1002/14651858.CD008409.pub3

[6] Sahuquillo J. Decompressive craniectomy for the treatment of refractory high intracranial pressure in traumatic brain injury. In: The Cochrane Collaboration, editor. Cochrane Database of Systematic Reviews. Chichester, UK: John Wiley & Sons, Ltd; 2006. [Internet]. [cited 2015 Dec 26]. Available from: http://doi.wiley.com/10.1002/14651858.CD003983.pub2

[7] National Institute of Neurological Disorders and Stroke. National Institute of Health - Traumatic Brain Injury. Traumatic Brain Injury; 2012

[8] MeSH. Neuroprotective Agents. Internet Based Definitions: NCBI. 1995. Available from: http://www.ncbi.nlm.nih.gov/mesh/68018696

[9] Burns TC, Verfaillie CM. From mice to mind: Strategies and progress in translating neuroregeneration. European Journal of Pharmacology. 2015;**759**:90-100

[10] Wright DW, Yeatts SD, Silbergleit R, Palesch YY, Hertzberg VS, Frankel M, et al. Very early administration of progesterone for acute traumatic brain injury. The New England Journal of Medicine. 2014;**371**(26):2457-2466

[11] Skolnick BE, Maas AI, Narayan RK, van der Hoop RG, MacAllister T, Ward JD, et al. A clinical trial of progesterone for severe traumatic brain injury. The New England Journal of Medicine. 2014; **371**(26):2467-2476

[12] Leucht S, Helfer B, Gartlehner G, Davis JM. How effective are common medications—A perspective based on meta-analyses of major drugs. BioMed Centeral Ltd—BMC Medicine. 2015; **13**(1):253

[13] Bracken MB. Steroids for acute spinal cord injury. Cochrane Database of Systematic Reviews. 2002. [Internet]. [cited 2015 Dec 26];3(3). Available

from: http://info.onlinelibrary.wiley.com/userfiles/ccoch/file/CD001046.pdf

[14] Atif F, Sayeed I, Ishrat T, Stein DG. Progesterone with vitamin D affords better neuroprotection against excitotoxicity in cultured cortical neurons than progesterone alone. Molecular Medicine. 2009;**15**(9–10):328

[15] Hoffmann S, Beyer C. Gonadal steroid hormones as therapeutic tools for brain trauma: The time is ripe for more courageous clinical trials to get into emergency medicine. The Journal of Steroid Biochemistry and Molecular Biology. 2015;**146**:1-2

[16] Robertson CL, Fidan E, Stanley RM, Noje C, Bayir H. Progesterone for neuroprotection in pediatric traumatic brain injury. Pediatric Critical Care Medicine. 2015;**16**(3):236-244

[17] Kelley BG, Mermelstein PG. Progesterone blocks multiple routes of ion flux. Molecular and Cellular Neurosciences. 2011;**48**(2):137-141

[18] Luoma JI, Kelley BG, Mermelstein PG. Progesterone inhibition of voltage-gated calcium channels is a potential neuroprotective mechanism against excitotoxicity. Steroids. 2011. [Internet]. [cited 2015 Dec 26]; Available from: http://linkinghub.elsevier.com/retrieve/pii/S0039128X11000535

[19] Forsyth RJ, Jayamoni B, Paine TC, Mascarenhas S. Monoaminergic agonists for acute traumatic brain injury. Cochrane Database of Systematic Reviews. Chichester, UK: John Wiley & Sons, Ltd; 2006. [Internet]. [cited 2015 Dec 26]. Available from: http://doi.wiley.com/10.1002/14651858.CD003984.pub2

[20] Abrishamkar S, Safavi M, Honarmand A. Effect of erythropoietin on Glasgow coma scale and Glasgow outcome Sale in patient with diffuse axonal injury. Journal of Research in Medical Sciences. 2012;**17**(1):51

[21] Nichol A, French C, Little L, Haddad S, Presneill J, Arabi Y, et al. Erythropoietin in traumatic brain injury (EPO-TBI): A double-blind randomised controlled trial. The Lancet. 2015; **386**(10012):2499-2506

[22] Presneill J, Little L, Nichol A, French C, Cooper D, Haddad S, et al. Statistical analysis plan for the erythropoietin in traumatic brain injury trial: A randomised controlled trial of erythropoietin versus placebo in moderate and severe traumatic brain injury. Trials. 2014;**15**(1):501

[23] Vink R, Cook NL, van den Heuvel C. Magnesium in acute and chronic brain injury: An update. Magnesium Research. 2009;**22**(3):158-162

[24] Wong GKC, Zhu XL, Poon WS. Beneficial effect of cerebrolysin on moderate and severe head injury patients: Result of a cohort study. In: Intracranial Pressure and Brain Monitoring XII. Springer; 2005. [Internet]. [cited 2015 Dec 26]. p. 59–60. Available from: http://link.springer.com/chapter/10.1007/3-211-32318-X_13

[25] Tan HB, Wasiak J, Rosenfeld JV, O'Donohoe TJ, Gruen RL. Citicoline (CDP-choline) for traumatic brain injury. In: The Cochrane Collaboration, editor. Cochrane Database of Systematic Reviews. Chichester, UK: John Wiley & Sons, Ltd; 2014. [Internet]. [cited 2015 Dec 26]. Available from: http://doi.wiley.com/10.1002/14651858.CD011217

[26] Chen C, Venketasubramanian N, Gan RN, Lambert C, Picard D, Chan BP, et al. Danqi Piantang Jiaonang (DJ), a traditional Chinese medicine, in poststroke recovery. Stroke. 2009; **40**(3):859-863

[27] Heurteaux C, Gandin C, Borsotto M, Widmann C, Brau F, Lhuillier M, et al. Neuroprotective and neuroproliferative activities of NeuroAid (MLC601,

MLC901), a Chinese medicine, in vitro and in vivo. Neuropharmacology. 2010; **58**(7):987-1001

[28] Mazzeo AT, Alves ÓL, Gilman CB, Hayes RL, Tolias C, Niki Kunene K, et al. Brain metabolic and hemodynamic effects of cyclosporin a after human severe traumatic brain injury: A microdialysis study. Acta Neurochirurgica. 2008;**150**(10): 1019-1031

[29] Mazzeo AT, Brophy GM, Gilman CB, Alves ÓL, Robles JR, Hayes RL, et al. Safety and tolerability of cyclosporin a in severe traumatic brain injury patients: Results from a prospective randomized trial. Journal of Neurotrauma. 2009;**26**(12):2195-2206

[30] Silver JM, Koumaras B, Chen M, Mirski D, Potkin SG, Reyes P, et al. Effects of rivastigmine on cognitive function in patients with traumatic brain injury. Neurology. 2006;**67**(5): 748-755

[31] Silver JM, Koumaras B, Meng X, Potkin SG, Reyes PF, Harvey PD, et al. Long-term effects of rivastigmine capsules in patients with traumatic brain injury. Brain Injury. 2009;**23**(2): 123-132

[32] Higgins J, Green S. Cochrane Handbook for Systematic Reviews of Interventions Version 5.1.0. 2011. Available from: http://handbook.cochrane.org

[33] Higgins JP, Thompson SG, Deeks JJ, Altman DG. Measuring inconsistency in meta-analyses. British Medical Journal. 2003;**327**(7414):557

[34] Rognås L, Hansen TM, Kirkegaard H, Tønnesen E. Anaesthesiologist-provided prehospital airway management in patients with traumatic brain injury: An observational study. European Journal of Emergency Medicine. 2014;**21**(6):418-423

[35] Bell MJ, Adelson PD, Hutchison JS, Kochanek PM, Tasker RC, Vavilala MS, et al. Differences in medical therapy goals for children with severe traumatic brain injury—An international study. Pediatric Critical Care Medicine. 2013; **14**(8):811-818

[36] Huizenga JE, Zink BJ, Maio RF, Hill EM. Guidelines for the management of severe head injury: Are emergency physicians following them? Academic Emergency Medicine. 2002;**9**(8): 806-812

[37] Cifu DX, Hart BB, West SL, Walker W, Carne W. The effect of hyperbaric oxygen on persistent postconcussion symptoms. The Journal of Head Trauma Rehabilitation. 2014;**29**(1):11-20

[38] Cifu DX, Walker WC, West SL, Hart BB, Franke LM, Sima A, et al. Hyperbaric oxygen for blast-related postconcussion syndrome: Three-month outcomes: HBO_2 RCT for PCS outcomes. Annals of Neurology. 2014;**75**(2): 277-286

[39] Cifu DX, Hoke KW, Wetzel PA, Wares JR, Gitchel G, Carne W. Effects of hyperbaric oxygen on eye tracking abnormalities in males after mild traumatic brain injury. Journal of Rehabilitation Research and Development. 2014;(7):51, 1047-1056

[40] Wolf G, Cifu D, Baugh L, Carne W, Profenna L. The effect of hyperbaric oxygen on symptoms after mild traumatic brain injury. Journal of Neurotrauma. 2012;**29**(17):2606-2612

[41] Wolf EG, Prye J, Michaelson R, Brower G, Profenna L, Boneta O. Hyperbaric side effects in a traumatic brain injury randomized clinical trial. [Internet]. DTIC Document; 2012 [cited 2015 Dec 26]. Available from: http://oai.dtic.mil/oai/oai?verb=getRecord&metadataPrefix=html&identifier=ADA611409

[42] Boussi-Gross R, Golan H, Fishlev G, Bechor Y, Volkov O, Bergan J, et al. Hyperbaric oxygen therapy can improve post concussion syndrome years after mild traumatic brain injury-randomized prospective trial. Ai J, editor. PLoS One. 2013;**8**(11):e79995

[43] Rockswold SB, Gaylan L, Rockswold DA, Jiannong L. A prospective, randomized phase II clinical trial to evaluate the effect of combined hyperbaric and normobaric hyperoxia on cerebral metabolism, intracranial pressure, oxygen toxicity, and clinical outcome in severe traumatic brain injury. Journal of Neurosurgery. 2013; **118**(6):1317-1328

[44] Shakeri M, Boustani MR, Pak N, Panahi F, Salehpour F, Lotfinia I, et al. Effect of progesterone administration on prognosis of patients with diffuse axonal injury due to severe head trauma. Clinical Neurology and Neurosurgery. 2013;**115**(10):2019-2022

[45] Wright DW, Kellermann AL, Hertzberg VS, Clark PL, Frankel M, Goldstein FC, et al. ProTECT: A randomized clinical trial of progesterone for acute traumatic brain injury. Annals of Emergency Medicine. 2007;**49**(4): 391-402.e2

[46] Xiao G, Wei J, Yan W, Wang W, Lu Z. Improved outcomes from the administration of progesterone for patients with acute severe traumatic brain injury: A randomized controlled trial. Critical Care. 2008;**12**(2):R61

[47] Wright DW, Ritchie JC, Mullins RE, Kellermann AL, Denson DD. Steady-state serum concentrations of progesterone following continuous intravenous infusion in patients with acute moderate to severe traumatic brain injury. Journal of Clinical Pharmacology. 2005;**45**(6):640-648

[48] Xiao G, Wei J, Wu Z, Wang W, Jiang Q, Cheng J, et al. Clinical study on the therapeutic effects and mechanism of progesterone in the treatment for acute severe head injury. Zhonghua Wai Ke Za Zhi. 2007;**45**(2):106-108

[49] Mammis A, McIntosh TK, Maniker AH. Erythropoietin as a neuroprotective agent in traumatic brain injury. Surgical Neurology. 2009;**71**(5):527-531

[50] Talving P, Lustenberger T, Kobayashi L, Inaba K, Barmparas G, Schnüriger B, et al. Erythropoiesis stimulating agent administration improves survival after severe traumatic brain injury: A matched case control study. Annals of Surgery. 2010;**251**(1): 1-4

[51] Aloizos S, Evodia E, Gourgiotis S, Isaia E, Seretis C, Baltopoulos G. Neuroprotective effects of erythropoietin in patients with severe closed brain injury. Turkish Neurosurgery. 2015. [Internet]. [cited 2015 Dec 26]; Available from: http://www.turkishneurosurgery.org.tr/summary_en_doi.php3?doi=10.5137/1019-5149.JTN.9685-14.4

[52] Natale JE, Guerguerian A-M, Joseph JG, McCarter R, Shao C, Slomine B, et al. Pilot study to determine the hemodynamic safety and feasibility of magnesium sulfate infusion in children with severe traumatic brain injury. Pediatric Critical Care Medicine. 2007; **8**(1):1-9

[53] Chen C-C, Wei S-T, Tsaia S-C, Chen X-X, Cho D-Y. Cerebrolysin enhances cognitive recovery of mild traumatic brain injury patients: Double-blind, placebo-controlled, randomized study. British Journal of Neurosurgery. 2013; **27**(6):803-807

[54] Poon W, Vos P, Muresanu D, Vester J, von Wild K, Hömberg V, et al. Cerebrolysin Asian Pacific trial in acute brain injury and neurorecovery: Design and methods. Journal of Neurotrauma. 2015;**32**(8):571-580

[55] Leon-Carrion J, Dominguez-Roldan J, Murillo-Cabezas F, del Rosario D, Munoz-Sanchez M. The role of citicholine in neuropsychological training after traumatic brain injury. Neuropsychological Rehabilitation. 1999;**14**(1):33-40

[56] Maldonado V, Perez J, Escario J. Effects of CDP-choline on the recovery of patients with head injury. Journal of the Neurological Sciences. 1991;**103**: 15-18

[57] Shokouhi G, Ghorbani Haghjoo A, Sattarnezhad N, Asghari M, Sattarnezhad A, Asghari A, et al. Effects of citicoline on level of consciousness, serum level of fetuin-A and matrix Gla-protein (MGP) in trauma patients with diffuse axonal injury (DAI) and GCS ≤ 8. Turkish Journal of Trauma and Emergency. 2014;**20**(6):410-416

[58] Zafonte RD, Bagiella E, Ansel B, Novack TA, Friedewald WT, Hesdorffer DC, et al. Effect of citicoline on functional and cognitive status among patients with traumatic brain injury: Citicoline brain injury treatment trial (COBRIT). Journal of the American Medical Association. 2012;**308**(19): 1993-2000

[59] Brophy GM, Mazzeo AT, Brar S, Alves OL, Bunnell K, Gilman C, et al. Exposure of Cyclosporin A in whole blood, cerebral spinal fluid, and brain extracellular fluid dialysate in adults with traumatic brain injury. Journal of Neurotrauma. 2013;**30**(17):1484-1489

[60] Empey PE, McNamara PJ, Young B, Rosbolt MB, Hatton J. Cyclosporin A disposition following acute traumatic brain injury. Journal of Neurotrauma. 2006;**23**(1):109-116

[61] Hatton J, Rosbolt B, Empey P, Kryscio R, Young B. Dosing and safety of cyclosporine in patients with severe brain injury: Clinical article. Journal of Neurosurgery. 2008;**109**(4):699-707

[62] Tenovuo O. Central acetylcholinesterase inhibitors in the treatment of chronic traumatic brain injury—Clinical experience in 111 patients. Progress in Neuro-Psychopharmacology & Biological Psychiatry. 2005;**29**(1):61-67

[63] Xu G-Z, Wang M-D, Liu K-G, Bai Y-A, Wu W, Li W. A meta-analysis of treating acute traumatic brain injury with calcium channel blockers. Brain Research Bulletin. 2013; **99**:41-47

[64] Cheng G, Fu L, Zhang H, Wang Y, Zhang L, Zhang J. The role of mitochondrial calcium uniporter in neuroprotection in traumatic brain injury. Medical Hypotheses. 2013;**80**(2): 115-117

[65] Hart T, Benn EKT, Bagiella E, Arenth P, Dikmen S, Hesdorffer DC, et al. Early trajectory of psychiatric symptoms after traumatic brain injury: Relationship to patient and injury characteristics. Journal of Neurotrauma. 2014;**31**(7):610-617

[66] Neumann D, Babbage DR, Zupan B, Willer B. A randomized controlled trial of emotion recognition training after traumatic brain injury. The Journal of Head Trauma Rehabilitation. 2015; **30**(3):E12-E23

[67] Li J, Jiang J. Chinese head trauma data bank: Effect of hyperthermia on the outcome of acute head trauma patients. Journal of Neurotrauma. 2012;**29**(1): 96-100

[68] Galvin IM, Levy R, Boyd JG, Day AG, Wallace MC. Cooling for cerebral protection during brain surgery. In: The Cochrane Collaboration, editor. Cochrane Database of Systematic Reviews [Internet]. Chichester, UK: John Wiley & Sons, Ltd; 2015. [cited 2015 Dec 26]. Available from: http://doi.wiley.com/10.1002/14651858.CD006638.pub3

[69] Maleki M, Ghaderi M, Ashktorab T, Jabbari-Noghabi H, Zadehmohammadi A. Effect of light music on physiological parameters of patients with traumatic brain injuries at intensive care unit. Ofogh-E-Danesh. 2011;**18**(1):66-75

[70] Nott M, Baguley I, Heriseanu R, Weber G, Middleton J, Meares S, et al. Effects of concomitant spinal cord injury and brain injury on medical and functional outcomes and community participation. Topics in Spinal Cord Injury Rehabilitation. 2014;**20**(3): 225-235

[71] Stein DG, Cekic MM. Progesterone and vitamin D hormone as a biologic treatment of traumatic brain injury in the aged. PM & R Journal. 2011;**3**(6): S100-S110

[72] Godbolt AK, Stenberg M, Jakobsson J, Sorjonen K, Krakau K, Stålnacke B-M, et al. Subacute complications during recovery from severe traumatic brain injury: Frequency and associations with outcome. BMJ Open. 2015;**5**(4):e007208

[73] Cinotti R, Ichai C, Orban J, Kalfon P, Feuillet F, Roquilly A, et al. Effects of tight computerized glucose control on neurological outcome in severely brain injured patients a multicenter sub-group analysis of the randomized-controlled open-label CGAO-REA study. Critical Care (London, England). 2014;**18**(5): 498

[74] Rhind SG, Crnko NT, Baker AJ, Morrison LJ, Shek PN, Scarpelini S, et al. Prehospital resuscitation with hypertonic saline-dextran modulates inflammatory, coagulation and endothelial activation marker profiles in severe traumatic brain injured patients. Journal of Neuroinflammation. 2010; 7(5):1-17

[75] Menon DK. Unique challenges in clinical trials in traumatic brain injury. Critical Care Medicine. 2009;**37** (Supplement):S129-S135

Chapter 6

Direct Brain Cooling in Treating Severe Traumatic Head Injury

Zamzuri Idris, Ang Song Yee, Regunath Kandasamy, Asrulnizam Abd Manaf, Mohd Hasyizan Bin Hassan and Wan Nazaruddin Wan Hassan

Abstract

There are scientific evidences that hypothermia provides a strong neuroprotective effect on the brain following traumatic insults. In this chapter, we describe the pathophysiology of severe head injury with emphasis on benefits of hypothermia. To support these hypothetical or theoretical benefits, we describe our previous study with very encouraging findings done on severe head injuries, treated with direct focal brain cooling, and monitored with intracranial pressure, cerebral perfusion pressure, brain oxygenation, and brain temperature. This chapter ends with our current and still ongoing study in which one of its main objectives is to innovate a direct focal brain cooling machine. This chapter briefly explains the technical part of this cooling machine.

Keywords: hypothermia, trauma, brain oxygenation, brain temperature, intracranial pressure, severe head injury, focal brain cooling

1. Introduction

Severe traumatic brain injury (TBI) is one of the causes contributed to the major source of death and severe disability worldwide. In some countries, the increasing number of severe traumatic brain injury is alarming, bringing negative impact not just toward the individual itself, but also the society. Patients suffering from severe traumatic brain injury usually will end up with disability, as they most often are associated with extensive irreversible damages to the brain. This makes the management of severe TBI to be challenging and very often associate with disappointing outcomes. Thus, severe TBI has become a common issue or interest that requires appropriate attention from various levels in order to reduce the damage impacts often associated with it. Many clinical trials and researches were conducted to improve our understanding and knowledge, with various treatment protocols being updated from time to time [1, 2].

During the trauma impact itself, there will be energy transfer to the brain tissue causing direct neuronal damages, causing irreversible damages to the neuronal structures, and affecting the neurophysiological function of the central nervous system. From the initial impact, primary injuries occur due to the direct impact and the damage that are usually irreversible. Secondary injuries will be subsequently triggered by hypoxic-ischemic event, inflammatory cytokines, and free radicals, which are released by the injured neuronal cells. Secondary injuries play an important role in determining posttraumatic recovery [3–5]. Secondary injuries will lead to breakdown of the cerebral blood brain barrier, leading to worsening cerebral edema and thus forming a vicious cycle toward further neuronal damages.

The management of severe TBI is aiming for restoration and maintenance of adequate brain perfusion to prevent hypoxia, surgical intervention for significant size of hematoma or edema, and prevention or prompt treatment of cerebral edema and raised intracranial pressure (ICP). However, clinical studies and analysis had proven that ICP and cerebral perfusion pressure (CPP) guided treatment alone, does not necessarily prevent hypoxic-ischemic damage to the brain [6]. Despite knowing that ICP remains the most important determinant factors of mortality outcome in severe head injury patients, brain hypoxia (defined as $PbtiO_2 < 10$ mmHg and for more than 15 minutes) is actually more important in determining the morbidity and patient functional outcome [7].

Many new strategies and alternative protocols are introduced to improve the management and outcome of severe TBI patients. Throughout the years, the definition of adequate cerebral resuscitation including the targeted ICP and CPP values are often debatable. Other treatment strategy such as $PbtiO_2$, plus ICP and CPP guided therapy showed promising result, with reduced hypoxic-ischemic damages to the brain and better patient functional outcome recovery.

Controlled systemic hypothermia treatment in managing severe head injury patient, is associated with neuroprotective effect to the injured brain tissue. Hypothermia significantly reduce metabolic rate and energy expenditure, attenuate excitatory amino acids and the synthesis of free radicals, suppresses excessive ischemia-induced and posttraumatic inflammatory reactions, and prevent blood-brain barrier disruption and brain edema. Furthermore, hyperthermia in head injury increases postischemic injury and is a significant predictor of poor outcome. Induced and controlled systemic hypothermia is used in patient with stroke, perinatal asphyxia, hypoxic encephalopathy following cardiovascular arrest with improved recovery, and functional outcome documented [8–11]. However, the pitfall of the treatment is that it is associated with alteration of the body core temperature and hence induced alteration in the systemic function and affecting the whole body hemostasis. Few possible adverse systemic complications that are associated with induced systemic hypothermia treatment include increase risk of infection and sepsis, pneumonia, poor wound healing and breakdown, cardiac arrhythmias, coagulopathy and electrolytes imbalances such as hypoglycemia and hypokalemia [12–18]. These systemic complications may outweigh the beneficial effect of the hypothermia treatment. Thus, treatment with induced and controlled systemic cooling therapy in head injury patient has become an interesting but controversial subject. Given so much controversy in inducing hypothermia for the injured brain, we sought to design a prospective, randomized pilot study to assess efficacy of new method in brain cooling called "direct regional or focal brain hypothermia." In this chapter, we present our experience with direct focal or regional brain cooling, obtained via direct irrigation of cold fluid onto the surface of severely injured brain of trauma patients who required decompressive craniectomy with Glasgow Coma Score (GCS) of 6–7, and the chapter ends with our current and still ongoing study in which, one of its main objectives is to innovate a direct focal brain cooling machine.

2. Role of hypothermia in head injury patient

There have been multiple mechanisms suggesting benefit of hypothermia in head injury patient. However, there is likely that no single factor can be used to explain the neuroprotective effect of hypothermia. Understanding the combination of the factors may help us understand better the effect of hypothermia [3]. The proposed mechanisms are summarized below [12, 19, 20] and depicted as in **Figure 1**.

a. Hypothermia can inhibit the activation of caspase enzymes.

b. It prevents or mitigates mitochondrial dysfunction.

c. It decreases the metabolism as well as decreases the overload of excitatory neurotransmitters such as glutamate and free oxygen radicals.

d. It modifies the cellular disorders of intracellular ion concentrations.

e. It suppresses the inflammatory and immunological responses and epileptic activity.

f. It reduces the disruption in blood brain barrier (BBB), vascular permeability, and edema.

g. It improves the microcirculatory circuits and intra- and extracellular acidosis.

h. It corrects the hyperthermia after brain injury and influences the local secretion of various vasoactive mediators secreted by the endothelium.

i. It enhances expression of immediate early genes and cold shock proteins.

j. Hypothermia may also influence neurogenesis, gliogenesis, and angiogenesis.

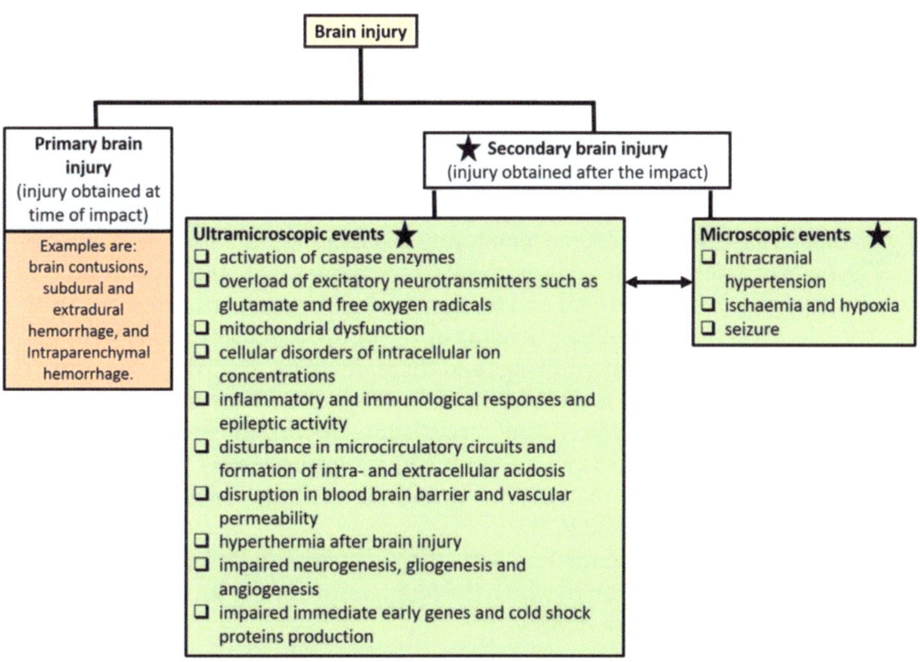

Figure 1.
Effect of hypothermia on pathophysiology of brain injury. Therapeutic hypothermia works by reducing the detrimental consequence of secondary brain injury (black stars).

3. Current evidences on the usage of direct brain cooling in treating severe head injury: animal studies

There are previously multiple papers that suggested targeted brain cooling as a reasonable treatment option to patient with severe traumatic brain injury [21–33]. Targeted brain cooling is a good alternative to systemic hypothermia, as systemic hypothermia has serious side effects such as circulatory constrain, increased risk of infection, electrolyte imbalance, and coagulopathy [15–18].

Jacek et al. [33] suggested in their animal study that selective brain hypothermia, which is applied via a cranial window after decompressive craniectomy seems to be reducing posttraumatic structural and functional damage. However, the study is actually limited by small rodent model and also short observational period. It is suggested that thermodynamic of brain of human rodent may differ as the size is significantly different. It may affect the penetration of the cooling effect in human brain, hence limiting the cooling effect to the superficial areas only.

4. Current evidences on the usage of direct brain cooling in treating severe head injury: our clinical study

Here, we describe our pilot study on direct focal hypothermia therapy in treating severe head injury with positive and very encouraging results that enable us to proceed with another innovative study to create a direct hypothermia machine, which will be used in our ongoing study.

4.1 Methodology

This is a randomized controlled trial study, which is designed to answer the research questions regarding the effect of direct focal brain cooling treatment in severe head injury patients. The study has been approved by the research and ethics committee and is sponsored by the Research University Grant. Patients were randomized into two treatment groups of A and B. Group B is the control group.

Group A (treatment group) consists of patients, who have therapy with direct focal brain cooling. All patients have intracranial pressure monitoring, Licox (focal brain oxygenation and temperature) probes inserted, and blood for immunological parameters. The immunological blood parameters are however taken only prior and after local cooling therapy to the brain. The overall monitoring and therapy period was for 48 hours.

The neurosurgical operations are standard operations, decompressive craniectomy covering frontal, parietal and temporal lobes; intracranial pressure probe insertion into the ventricle or parenchyma of the brain, and Licox probe into abnormal brain areas. The monitorings and therapies given after the surgery are the standard therapy for severe head injury patient (**Figure 2**). They include sedation with or without muscle paralysis agents, ventilator support, hypertonic saline or mannitol, draining of cerebrospinal fluid (CSF) for the persistent raise in intracranial pressure (ICP) of more than 20 mmHg and thiopentone coma therapy as a final step to treat persistently raised ICP.

Direct focal brain cooling method done through persistently irrigating the brain with cold Hartmann's solution in which the temperature of the infused fluid is divided into two subgroups as follow:

1. Deep cooling: temperature of 20–29°C.

2. Mild cooling: temperature of 30–36°C.

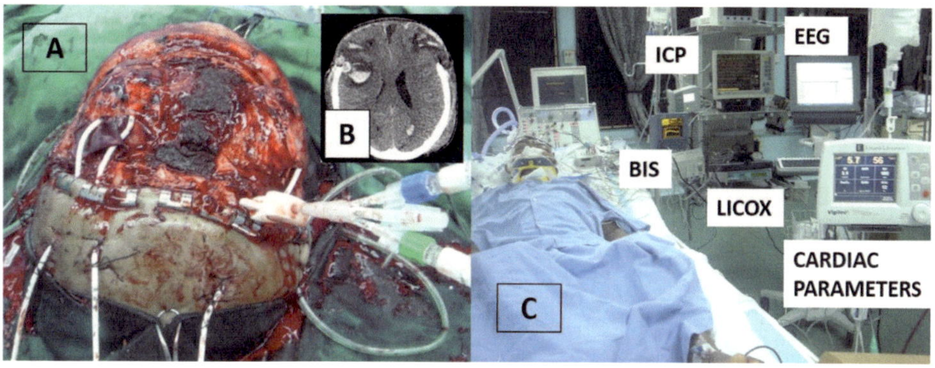

Figure 2.
Direct brain cooling monitoring and therapy. (A) intraoperative bifrontal decompressive craniectomy with insertion of Licox and ICP probes; (B) inset image: Post-op CT scan; (C) neurointensive care management and monitorings with Licox, cardiac parameters, ICP, bispectral index (BIS) and electroencephalography (EEG).

The Hartmann's solution was infused via Neurojaf external ventricular drainage (EVD) catheter, which was inserted superior to the dura flap and at the inner surface of the dura, acting like rains flushing through the surface of the swollen brain (multiple extra holes are made). The catheter is in contact with the surface of the brain. The infusion rate is 70 mls/hr. Due to the position of the head, the second draining tube will be inserted at the lower part of the craniectomy flap outside the dura (which is closed loosely) to drain the excess fluid with low suction pressure. The temperature of the infused Hartmann's solution is checked via the three-way connector draining the fluid out to the collection port for temperature assessment. If temperature reading is under or above the intended value, new solution with correct intended temperature will replace the previous one.

All patients will have CT scan done if the ICP shows persistently raised values despite of standard therapies given. This is important to exclude any new surgical lesion and to exclude the retention of infused solution as a cause of raised ICP. If

	No cooling	**Mild cooling**	**Deep cooling**	**Total**
Total patients	13	10	9	32
Variables	No cooling	Mild cooling	Deep cooling	P value
Age (mean in years) [95% CI]	45.5 [35.0–56.1]	28.9 [17.3–40.5]	26.7 [11.9–41.4]	0.02
Gender (number):				
1. Male	10	8	9	
2. Female	3	2	0	0.40
GCS (median)	6	7	7	0.38
Injury Severity Score (mean) [95% CI]	27.8 [21.2–34.5]	24.0 [18.5–29.5]	28.7 [21.3–36.0]	0.56
Marshall Score (median)	4	4	3	0.33
Patients with disseminated intravascular coagulopathy (DIVC)	3	2	4	0.44

Table 1.
Basic parameters comparison among three studied groups.

the ICPs show normal values, the CT scan of the brain is done after 48 hours of therapy prior to removal of the EVD tube to document the location of the EVD tip. The measured outcomes are: (a) trend and values for monitored parameters (ICPs, CPPs, brain temperature and focal brain oxygenation), (b) Glasgow Outcome Score (GOS – good and poor GOS), and (c) immunological parameters.

4.2 Results

4.2.1 Social demographic data of patients included in the study

There were 32 patients recruited in this study with 27 male patients and 5 female patients. The median age of patients recruited were 45.5 in no cooling group, whereas 28.9 and 26.7, respectively, for mild cooling and deep cooling groups. Median GCS for the patients recruited were 6–7. The highest injury severity score recruited was 36, whereas the lowest was 18.5. The median Marshall score for patient recruited were 3–4. Patients with disseminated intravascular coagulopathy for no cooling, mild cooling, and deep cooling were 3, 2, and 4 patients, respectively. The demographic data is shown in **Table 1**.

4.2.2 Effects of direct focal brain cooling on median ICP, CPP, brain oxygenation, and temperature

The trend of the ICPs, CPPs, brain temperature, and focal brain oxygenation for all studied groups are shown in **Figure 3A–D**. During 48 hours of observation and monitoring, there is no significant statistical difference in overall 4 hourly mean ICPs, CPPs, and brain temperature amongst the no cooling, mild cooling, and deep cooling groups; but there is significant statistical difference in overall 4 hourly mean focal brain oxygenation according to repeated measure ANOVA (between groups analysis based on time) (depicted in **Tables 2** and **3**).

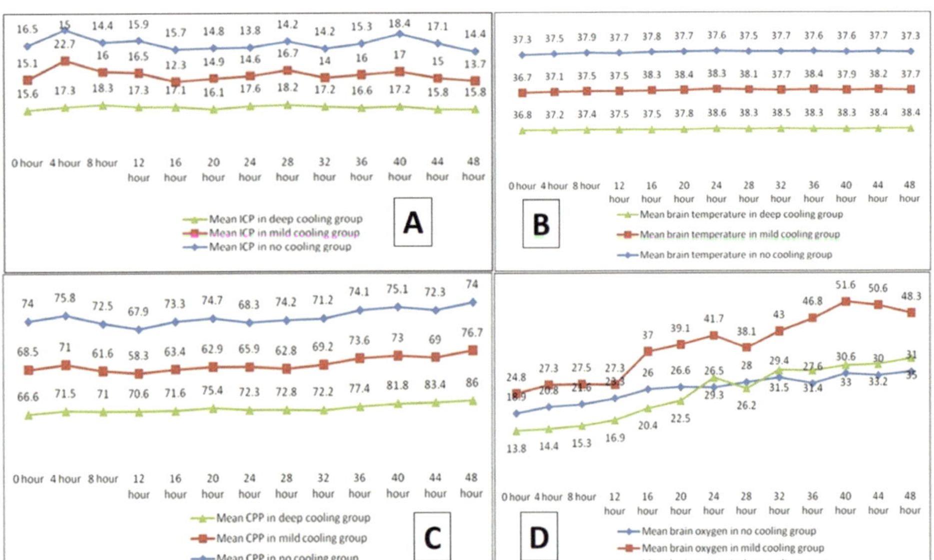

Figure 3.
(A) Trend of ICPs in the first 48 hours after the treatment. (B) Trend of brain temperature observation for the first 48 hours after treatment. (C) Trend of CPPs in the first 48 hours after the treatment. (D) Trend of brain oxygen observation for the first 48 hours after treatment.

Table 2 shows day 1 of monitoring and treatment, mean brain oxygenation of mild cooling group has mostly fallen outside the 95% CI (confidence interval) of deep cooling group. Therefore, there is significant difference in mean brain oxygen between mild cooling and deep cooling; with mild cooling having significantly higher mean brain oxygen values. On day 2 of monitoring and treatment, mean brain oxygenation of no cooling group has mostly also fallen outside the 95% CI of mild cooling group. Therefore, there is significant difference in mean brain oxygen between no cooling and mild cooling. Likewise to day one findings, there is also a significant difference on day 2 in mean brain oxygen between mild cooling and deep cooling. Interestingly, in all group comparisons, mild brain cooling group has significantly higher mean brain oxygenation values as compared to either deep or no cooling group (depicted in **Table 3**).

4.2.3 Effect of regional brain cooling on GOS at discharge and at 6 months

There is no significant difference in GOS at time of discharge for both studied groups (no cooling vs. cooling groups). However, there is significant difference on good GOS in cooling group compared to no cooling group at 6 months follow-up (as shown in **Table 4** with $p < 0.007$). On stratifying the cooling group further into deep and mild cooling, it shows that there is significant difference in term of GOS score at 6 months with significant better outcomes noted in mild cooling as compared to no cooling group with $p < 0.013$. The deep cooling group at 6 months outcome, failed to have significant difference value when compared with either no or mild cooling groups. For this reason, direct and mild brain hypothermia

Time (Day 1)	Treatment group	Mean brain oxygen	95% confidence interval (CI)
0 hour	No cooling	18.94	8.29–29.60
	Mild cooling	28.27	15.54–41.01
	Deep cooling	13.82	1.91–25.73
4 hour	No cooling	20.78	11.72–29.83
	Mild cooling	31.17	***20.35–41.99***
	Deep cooling	14.43	4.31–24.55
8 hour	No cooling	21.55	12.40–30.70
	Mild cooling	31.39	***20.45–42.32***
	Deep cooling	15.33	5.10–25.56
12 hour	No cooling	23.27	15.31–31.22
	Mild cooling	31.14	***21.64–40.65***
	Deep cooling	16.89	8.00–25.78
16 hours	No cooling	25.96	16.30–35.62
	Mild cooling	36.93	***25.38–48.47***
	Deep cooling	20.36	9.56–31.16
20 hours	No cooling	26.64	16.22–37.05
	Mild cooling	39.11	***26.67–51.56***
	Deep cooling	22.51	10.86–34.15

Statistical analysis: Repeated Measure ANOVA (between groups analysis based on time).

Table 2.
Comparison of mean brain oxygen between three treatment groups based on 4 hourly observations (day 1).

Time (Day 2)	Treatment group	Mean brain oxygen	95% confidence interval (CI)
0 hour	No cooling	28.00	16.98–39.03
	Mild cooling	48.73	31.89–65.58
	Deep cooling	28.91	14.32–43.49
4 hours	No cooling	29.20	16.98–41.43
	Mild cooling	50.17	***31.50–68.84***
	Deep cooling	28.13	11.96–44.30
8 hours	No cooling	28.96	17.57–40.35
	Mild cooling	52.27	***34.87–69.66***
	Deep cooling	34.39	19.33–49.46
12 hours	No cooling	27.46	18.63–36.30
	Mild cooling	52.00	***38.51–65.49***
	Deep cooling	33.69	22.01–45.38
16 hours	No cooling	30.63	21.34–39.92
	Mild cooling	51.60	***37.41–65.79***
	Deep cooling	35.17	22.88–47.45
20 hours	No cooling	30.05	20.01–40.08
	Mild cooling	50.57	***35.24–65.90***
	Deep cooling	36.12	22.84–49.39

Statistical analysis: Repeated Measure ANOVA (between groups analysis based on time).

Table 3.
Comparison of brain oxygen between three treatment groups based on 4 hourly observations (day 2).

with coolant temperature of 30–36°C might truly be beneficial to the severely head injured patients. Having said that, obviously future studies are still needed to ascertain this finding with higher number of more homogenous recruited patients.

4.2.4 Effects of regional brain cooling on immunological parameters

There is no significant difference on immunological parameters upon comparing prior and after cooling therapy. Nonetheless, the postcooling immunological parameters seem to have lower values than the precooling ones (depicted in **Table 5**).

4.3 Discussion

This was a randomized controlled pilot study involving 32 patients, who were admitted to our hospital with severe head injury with GCS of 6 or 7. The aim was to study the effect of direct focal brain cooling therapy in severe head injury patients.

4.3.1 Effect of direct focal brain cooling on brain oxygen level

All the treatment groups were able to reach the desired mean brain oxygen level within the treatment period. Notwithstanding, the mean brain oxygen of mild cooling group was significantly higher as compared to the no- and deep cooling groups. It remained significantly higher throughout the treatment periods (24–48 hours) with the level of >50 mmHg. The mean brain oxygen of deep cooling group was the

Outcomes (GOS)	**No cooling [13 patients]**	**Cooling group [19 patients]**		**p value**
Poor GOS (GOS 1–3)				
Good GOS (GOS 4–5)				
Comparing 2 groups				
GOS at discharge:				
a. Poor GOS	12 (92.3%)	15 (78.9%)		0.307
b. Good GOS	1 (7.7%)	4 (21.1%)		
GOS at 6 months:				
a. Poor GOS	11 (84.6%)	7 (36.8%)		**0.007***
b. Good GOS	2 (15.4%)	12 (63.2%)		
Comparing 3 groups	***No cooling [n (%)]***	***Mild cooling [n (%)]***	***Deep cooling [n (%)]***	
GOS at 6 months:				
a. Poor GOS	11(84.6%)	3 (30%)	4 (44.4%)	0.023*
b. Good GOS	2 (15.4%)	7 (70%)	5 (55.6%)	
GOS at 6 months:				
a. Poor GOS	11 (84.6%)	3 (30%)		0.013*
b. Good GOS	2 (15.4%)	7 (70%)		
GOS at 6 months:				
a. Poor GOS	11 (84.6%)		4 (44.4%)	0.074
b. Good GOS	2 (15.4%)		5 (55.6%)	
GOS at 6 months:				
a. Poor GOS		3 (30%)	4 (44.4%)	0.650
b. Good GOS		7 (70%)	5 (55.6%)	

**Statistically significant. Statistical analysis: Pearson Chi-squared test.*

Table 4.
Effect of regional brain cooling on GOS at discharge and at 6 months; and effect of regional brain cooling on GOS only at 6 months, after stratifying the cooling group further into mild and deep cooling.

lowest but still did not reach the critical ischemic state (10–15 mmHg). Despite of having the lowest brain oxygen level on day 1, the improvement in brain oxygen level in deep cooling group was accelerated and reached the desirable range after 16 hours of treatment (with mean brain oxygen of >20 mmHg).

Patients with severe head injury were at higher risk of developing cerebral ischemia particularly in the first 48 hours. Cerebral ischemia was defined by brain oxygen of <10 mmHg for more than 2 hours [34]. Low mean brain oxygen pressure often associated with poorer clinical outcome, while patients with good GOS often had good or normalized reading within 2 hours after the injury. Brain oxygen level is a good indicator of functional outcome in addition to ICP and CPP. Targeted therapy of ICP < 15 mmHg, CPP > 75 mmHg, and brain oxygen >25 mmHg often associated with good clinical outcomes. The clinical trials comparing the ICP-CPP guided therapy to ICP-CPP-brain oxygen guided therapy showed significant better functional outcome at 6 months and lower mortality rate in the latter group [34, 35]. This showed that ICP-CPP-brain oxygen guided therapy is beneficial in treating severe head injury patients as it can improve the patient outcomes.

	Precooling (mean ± SD)	Postcooling (mean ± SD)	Wilcoxon signed Ranked test (p value)
T-cell markers (cells/mm^3)			
CD 3	776.8 (407.5)	756.3 (339.9)	0.86
CD 4	443.1 (268.5)	429.7 (210.0)	0.64
CD 8	328.1 (183.6)	301.7 (135.7)	0.96
CD 19	284.4 (168.6)	261.5 (126.6)	0.62
CD 16 and 56	172.4 (113.8)	112.7 (80.8)	0.05
Pro-inflammatory cytokines (pg/ml)			
Interleukin-1 (IL-1)	45.34 (130.7)	5.7 (13.0)	0.33
Interleukin-6 (IL-6)	278.5 (221.1)	190.0 (208.4)	0.44
Tumor necrosis factor (TNF)	34.5 (37.6)	18.1 (14.2)	0.41
Other immunological parameters			
Total WBC	13.6 (5.0)	12.8 (4.0)	0.16

Table 5.
Effect of regional brain cooling (both mild and deep cooling groups combined together) on immunological parameters.

4.3.2 Effect of direct focal brain cooling on ICP and CPP

The mean ICP did not show any significant difference amongst the studied groups as shown in the results above. There was also no evidence of refractory intracranial hypertension throughout the treatment period in all three groups, indicating that the focal cooling therapy used in this study was safe and not associated with risk of intracranial hypertension. The results seemed to contradict the effect of hypothermia, which supposed to have better control on ICPs, and hence, leading to better CPPs and mean brain oxygenation. Previous clinical study on the effect of mild systemic hypothermia to the head injury patients clearly had established a significant reduction in ICPs following cooling therapy [36]. The mechanisms of reduction in ICP values were postulated to be due to reduced cerebral edema, following an improvement of:

1. the blood brain barrier [37],

2. vascular permeability of microvascular endothelial cells [38],

3. extravasation of hemoglobin [39],

4. membrane disintegration processes,

5. cytotoxic edema via decreased inflammatory reactions and free radical formation within the brain, and

6. ion homeostasis including calcium [40].

Reduction in ICP and improvement in CPP did not happen in our pilot study, perhaps, because decompressive craniectomy had been completed prior to direct hypothermia therapy. Hence, intracranial pressure and perfusion pressure effects might not be shown-up in this particular study. Nevertheless, future related study should be carried out with more homogenous patients to confirm this finding.

4.3.3 Effect of direct focal brain cooling on brain temperature

There was no significant difference in brain temperature in all treatment groups as shown above in trend-results, thus showing that focal cooling did not seem to be effective in reducing focal brain temperature. This study was initially designed to reduce brain temperature; the mechanism of temperature reduction was thought to be achieved through two ways, which were direct cooling effect over the brain surface (via continuous irrigation of the cold Hartmann fluid) as well as through the indirect cooling effect (to the deeper part of the brain) via circulation and pulsation around the brain and cisterns. However, it seemed that the targeted effect was not achieved. This can be due to many factors including poor CSF circulation, and hence affecting the thermoregulation of the brain. It is worth mentioning that there is limitation of Licox probe as well. This device was specifically designed to detect the changes occurred around the area where it was inserted. Hence, it was unable to reflect accurately the whole brain temperature changes following head injury [41].

It was well documented in the literature that an injured brain might have significantly higher temperature compared to the core body temperature; ranging from 0.1°C to more than 2°C. The difference in the temperature gradient may be more significant in an injured brain as a result of destructive hyperactivity of the injured cells [42]. Numerous clinical studies have found that higher brain temperature is associated with adverse outcome and negative correlation with the prognosis of head injury patients. Hyperthermia increases the risk of ischemic area to become necrotic or apoptotic. In animal model, transient increase in core body temperature to 39–40°C led to 2.6-fold increase in the extent of neuronal injury in the hippocampus [43]. Since hyperthermia was an important independent factor of adverse neurological outcome and increase mortality in brain injury [44], accurate brain temperature reading was rather essential. For future reference, focal brain temperature reading with Licox may be combined with adjunct devices such as CT thermography as it can accurately measure the focal and whole brain temperature for better comparison during treatment.

4.3.4 Effect of direct focal brain cooling on the Glasgow Outcome Score (GOS)

Patients GOS was the most important factor to determine the outcome of the focal brain cooling treatment in this study. This classification system was specifically designed to help clinicians to determine the patients response following the treatment by assessing their functional status at discharge and at 6 months after the injury; score 1 reflects mortality, score 2 and 3 reflect significant morbidity, while score 4 and 5 reflect ability to function normally or near normal. The outcomes were promising as significant difference was noted, whereby the proportion of patients who received direct focal brain cooling treatment showed better GOS score of 4 and 5 at 6 months follow-up when compared to the no cooling group. However, no significant difference was established in GOS at day of discharge. The outcome of patient in severe head injury is actually multifactorial and could not just be attributed to a single factor. The age, other associated injuries, and hemodynamic instability will all contribute to the outcomes of the patients. The obvious contributing factor in our study is the increment in focal brain oxygenation during cooling therapy and it is markedly obvious in mild cooling group who received cold-fluid of 30–36°C.

4.3.5 Effect of direct focal brain cooling on immune responses

In this study, the T-cell markers, pro-inflammatory cytokines, and total white cell count show reduction in values after cooling therapy; nonetheless, no significant statistical difference noted in each studied immune parameters. This may be due to our small sample size; therefore, future related study should consider to recruit more patients with better homogenous participants' population. Besides this drawback, another shortcoming is no level taken from non-cooling group for comparison, thus the true effect of regional brain cooling on immunological biomarkers cannot be truly ascertained. This initial result, however, might indicate that focal brain cooling treatment has little adverse effect onto immune responses, which often associated with induced systemic cooling. Following head injury, acute immunological responses to the trauma begin around 1 hour after the injury until several days. Pro inflammatory mediators such as tumor necrosis factors-alpha (TNF-α) and IL-1 are released from injured tissues and stimulate the migration of the leukocytes across the BBB. These lead to accumulation of the inflammatory cells in the injured brain within hours. Activation of the complement systems following head injury will stimulate the neutrophil and in later stages, also monocytes and macrophages. These initial stages are basically causing granulocytosis (up to 90%), increasing immunoglobulins (Ig)-E, slight increase or normal level of monocytes, B-lymphocytes as well as Ig-A, -G and -M. On the other hand, there is suppression of the other lymphocytes subsets particularly the CD3, CD4 and CD8 counts [45]. Some of these changes were found to be beneficial and associated with neuroprotective effects while some other inflammatory mediators were neurotoxic [46]. The CD3, CD4, and CD8 counts are normally suppressed after few hours following severe head injury. This level will remain low for the next 24–48 hours and generally normalized after 3 days. The CD8 count tends to normalize faster than the CD3 and CD4. Increased risk of infection had been attributed to the suppression of these cellular immunities. Besides these mechanisms in causing alterations in immune parameters, other possibilities should also be considered. Those possibilities include:

1. blood product transfusion pre-, intra-, or postoperatively,

2. possibility of neuroendocrine changes,

3. the duration of the surgery,

4. the incidence of pre- and intraoperative hypothermia, which were not documented, and

5. the severity of trauma with consideration of the extend of tissues damaged [47].

5. Current innovation in direct focal brain cooling: D-Brain Cooling Machine™

The internal cooling methods use central venous catheters to either infuse cold saline or directly to reduce the blood temperature by convection. By advancement in microelectronic industry, instrumentation system can be integrated on chip level that can miniaturize the system to micro dimension. One of the advancements is miniaturization of micro-controller that can be easier to interface with sensing instrumentation system. Thus in this project, simple and intelligent localized brain cooling instrument by using Programmable System on Chip (PSoC) is proposed. Advantages of this system are simple, can localize coolant area in brain and System on chip (SoC) based automation system. This project involves designing temperature chamber to place the sterile fluid that is connected with antibiotic piping directly to

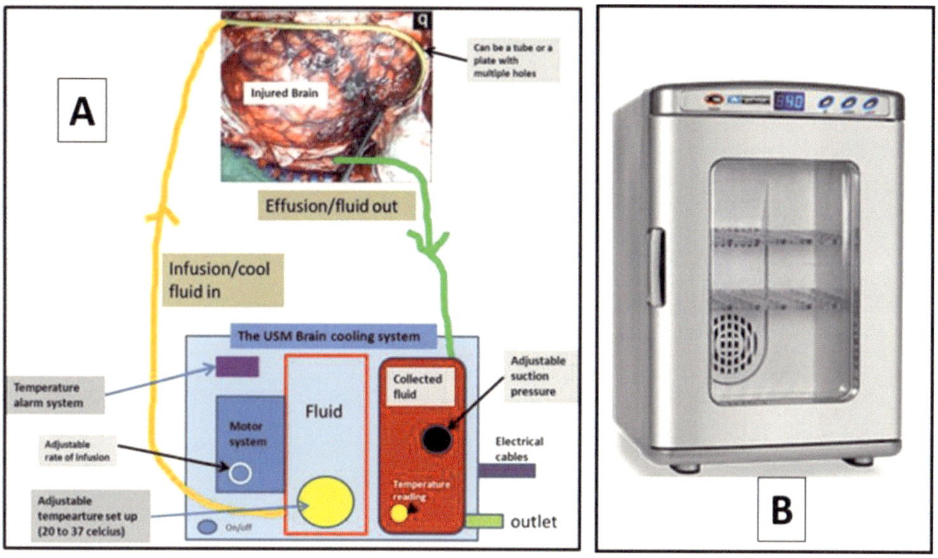

Figure 4.
Direct brain cooling or D-brain cooling machine™. (A) Its principles; and (B) Illustration of final image of adjustable temperature chamber.

the brain location. This chamber will be integrated with temperature controller, then, processed by PSoC microcontroller, as shown in **Figure 4A** and **B**. Subsequently, sensing and micro-controller will be interfaced to the system for temperature display. This direct brain cooling machine is known as D-Brain Cooling Machine™.

6. Conclusions

This chapter highlights the fascinating result of our pilot study on direct focal brain cooling therapy in severe head injury patients. The significant clinical outcome results seem in mild cooling group is thought to be due to an elevation in oxygenation level of injured and decompressed brain tissues. Thus, direct brain cooling therapy seems as a promising treatment in severe head injuries, and should be considered by neurosurgeon and neurointensivist as an adjunctive method to decompressive craniectomy. Therefore, combination of both therapies may help many diffused and severely injured brains secondary to neurotrauma in gaining better clinical outcomes. Base on this initial and encouraging results, there is ongoing study by our group on direct focal brain cooling therapy in severely head injured patients by using newly invented cooling machine named D-Brain cooling machine™ therapy.

Acknowledgements

This chapter was funded by Research University (RUi) Grant (Grant No. USM/JEPeM/18010074).

Conflict of interest

None declared.

Author details

Zamzuri Idris[1*], Ang Song Yee[1], Regunath Kandasamy[1], Asrulnizam Abd Manaf[2], Mohd Hasyizan Bin Hassan[3] and Wan Nazaruddin Wan Hassan[3]

1 Department of Neurosciences, School of Medical Sciences, Universiti Sains Malaysia, Kelantan, Malaysia

2 Collaborative Microelectronic Design Excellence Center (CEDEC), Engineering Campus Universiti Sains Malaysia, Nibong Tebal, Pulau Pinang, Malaysia

3 Neuroanaesthesia Division, School of Medical Sciences, Universiti Sains Malaysia, Kelantan, Malaysia

*Address all correspondence to: neuroscienceszamzuri@yahoo.com

References

[1] Narayan RK et al. Clinical trials in head injury. Journal of Neurotrauma. 2002;**19**(5):503-557

[2] Maas AIR et al. Re-orientation of clinical research in traumatic brain injury: Report of an international workshop on comparative effectiveness research. Journal of Neurotrauma. 2012;**29**(1):32-46

[3] Nortje J, Menon DK. Traumatic brain injury: Physiology, mechanisms, and outcome. Current Opinion in Neurology. 2004;**17**(6):711-718

[4] Farag E, Manno EM, Kurz A. Use of hypothermia for traumatic brain injury: Point of view. Minerva Anestesiologica. 2011;**77**(3):366-370

[5] Kurland D et al. Hemorrhagic progression of a contusion after traumatic brain injury: A review. Journal of Neurotrauma. 2012;**29**(1):19-31

[6] Stiefel MF, Udoetuk JD, Spiotta AM, Gracias VH, Goldberg A, Maloney-Wilenskey E, et al. Conventional neurocritical care and cerebral oxygenation after traumatic brain injury. Journal of Neurosurgery. 2006;**105**:568-575

[7] Maloney-Wilensky E, Gracias V, Itkin A, Hoffman K, Bloom S, Yang W, et al. Brain tissue oxygen and outcome after severe traumatic brain injury: A systematic review. Critical Care Medicine. 2009;**37**(6):2057-2063

[8] Corry JJ et al. Hypothermia for refractory status epilepticus. Neurocritical Care. 2008;**9**(2):189-197

[9] Gluckman PD et al. Selective head cooling with mild systemic hypothermia after neonatal encephalopathy: Multicentre randomised trial. Lancet. 2005;**365**(9460):663-670

[10] Jacobs S et al. Cooling for newborns with hypoxic ischaemic encephalopathy. Cochrane Database of Systematic Reviews. 2007;**4**:Cd003311

[11] Kramer C et al. Therapeutic hypothermia for severe traumatic brain injury: A critically appraised topic. The Neurologist. 2012;**18**(3):173-177

[12] Polderman KH. Application of therapeutic hypothermia in the intensive care unit. Opportunities and pitfalls of a promising treatment modality—Part 2: Practical aspects and side effects. Intensive Care Medicine. 2004;**30**(5):757-769

[13] Polderman KH, Herold I. Therapeutic hypothermia and controlled normothermia in the intensive care unit: Practical considerations, side effects, and cooling methods. Critical Care Medicine. 2009;**37**(3):1101-1120

[14] Peterson K, Carson S, Carney N. Hypothermia treatment for traumatic brain injury: A systematic review and meta-analysis. Journal of Neurotrauma. 2008;**25**(1):62-71

[15] Andrews PJ et al. Hypothermia for intracranial hypertension after traumatic brain injury. The New England Journal of Medicine. 2015;**373**(25):2403-2412

[16] Clifton GL, Miller ER, Sung CC, et al. Lack of effect of induction of hypothermia after acute brain injury. New England Journal of Medicine. 2001;**344**:556-563

[17] Shiozaki T et al. A multicenter prospective randomized controlled trial of the efficacy of mild hypothermia for severely head injured patients with low intracranial pressure. Mild Hypothermia Study Group in Japan. Journal of Neurosurgery. 2001;**94**(1):50-54

[18] O'Phelan KH et al. Therapeutic temperature modulation is associated with pulmonary complications in patients with severe traumatic brain injury. World Journal of Critical Care Medicine. 2015;**4**(4):296-301

[19] Yenari MA, Han HS. Neuroprotective mechanisms of hypothermia in brain ischaemia. Nature Reviews. Neuroscience. 2012;**13**(4):267-278

[20] Tripathy S, Mahapatra AK. Targeted temperature management in brain protection: An evidence-based review. Indian Journal of Anaesthesia. 2015;**59**(1):9-14

[21] Idris Z et al. Better Glasgow outcome score, cerebral perfusion pressure and focal brain oxygenation in severely traumatized brain following direct regional brain hypothermia therapy: A prospective randomized study. Asian Journal of Neurosurgery. 2014;**9**(3):115-123

[22] Kuluz J et al. Selective brain cooling during and after prolonged global ischemia reduces cortical damage in rats. Stroke. 1992;**23**:1792-1796; discussion 1797

[23] Tadler SC, Callaway CW, Menegazzi JJ. Noninvasive cerebral cooling in a swine model of cardiac arrest. Academic Emergency Medicine. 1998;**5**(1):25-30

[24] Gelman B et al. Selective brain cooling in infant piglets after cardiac arrest and resuscitation. Critical Care Medicine. 1996;**24**(6):1009-1017

[25] Kuluz JW et al. Selective brain cooling increases cortical cerebral blood flow in rats. The American Journal of Physiology. 1993;**265**(3 Pt 2):H824-H827

[26] Pil WH et al. Comparative neuroprotective efficacy of prolonged moderate intraischemic and postischemic hypothermia in focal cerebral ischemia. Journal of Neurosurgery. 2000;**92**(1):91-99

[27] Thoresen M et al. Effective selective head cooling during posthypoxic hypothermia in newborn piglets. Pediatric Research. 2001;**49**(4):594-599

[28] Doll H et al. Pharyngeal selective brain cooling is associated with reduced CNS cortical lesion after experimental traumatic brain injury in rats. Journal of Neurotrauma. 2010;**27**(12):2245-2254

[29] King C et al. Brain temperature profiles during epidural cooling with the ChillerPad in a monkey model of traumatic brain injury. Journal of Neurotrauma. 2010;**27**(10):1895-1903

[30] Cheng G et al. Effects of selective head cooling on cerebral blood flow and metabolism in newborn piglets after hypoxia-ischemia. Early Human Development. 2011;**87**(2):109-114

[31] Yao C et al. Selective brain cooling in rats ameliorates intracerebral hemorrhage and edema caused by penetrating brain injury: Possible involvement of heme oxygenase-1 expression. Journal of Neurotrauma. 2011;**28**(7):1237-1245

[32] Kim J-H et al. Delayed and prolonged local brain hypothermia combined with decompressive craniectomy: A novel therapeutic strategy that modulates glial dynamics. Experimental Neurobiology. 2014;**23**(2):115-123

[33] Szczygielski J et al. Selective brain hypothermia mitigates brain damage and improves neurological outcome after post-traumatic decompressive craniectomy in mice. Journal of Neurotrauma. 2017;**34**(8):1623-1635

[34] Narotam PK, Morrison JF, Nathoo N. Brain tissue oxygen monitoring in traumatic brain injury and major

trauma: Outcome analysis of a brain tissue oxygen-directed therapy. Journal of Neurosurgery. 2009;**111**:672-682

[35] Spiotta AM, Stiefel MF, Gracias VH, Garuffe AM, Kofke WA, Maloney-Wilensky E, et al. Brain tissue oxygen-directed management and outcome in patients with severe traumatic brain injury. Journal of Neurosurgery. 2010;**113**:571-580

[36] Polderman KH. Induced hypothermia and fever control for prevention and treatment of neurological injuries. Lancet Neurology. 2008;**371**:1955-1969

[37] Huang ZG, Xue D, Preston E, Karbalai H, Buchan AM. Biphasic opening of the blood-brain barrier following transient focal ischaemia: Effects of hypothermia. The Canadian Journal of Neurological Sciences. 1999;**26**:298-304

[38] Jurkovich GJ, Pitt RM, Curreri PW, Granger DN. Hypothermia prevents increased capillary permeability following ischaemia - reperfusion injury. Journal of Surgical Research. 1988;**44**:514-521

[39] Kinoshita K, Chatzipanteli K, Alonso OF, Howard M, Dietrich WD. The effect of brain temperature on hemoglobin extravasation after traumatic brain injury. Journal of Neurosurgery. 2002;**97**:945-953

[40] Fischer S, Renz D, Wiesnet M, Schaper W, Karliczek GF. Hypothermia abolishes hypoxia-induced hyperpermeability in brain microvessel endothelial cells. Brain Research. Molecular Brain Research. 1999;**74**:135-144

[41] Rabinstein AA. Elucidating the value of continuous brain oxygen monitoring. Neurocritical Care. 2010;**12**:144-145

[42] Henker RA, Brown SD, Marion DW. Comparison of brain temperature with bladder and rectal temperature in adults with severe head injury. Neurosurgery. 1998;**42**:1071-1075

[43] Baena RC, Busto R, Dietrich WD, Globus MY, Ginsberg MD. Hyperthermia delayed by 24 hours aggravates neuronal damage in rat hippocampus following global ischaemia. Neurology. 1997;**48**:768-773

[44] Hajat C, Hajat S, Sharma P. Effect of post stroke pyrexia on stroke outcome: A meta-analysis of studies on patients. Stroke. 2000;**31**:410-414

[45] Smrcka M, Mrlian A, Klabusay M. Immune system status in the patients after severe brain injury. Bratislavské Lekárske Listy. 2005;**106**(3):144-146

[46] Morganti-Kossmann MC, Rancan M, Stahel PF, Kossmann T. Inflammatory response in acute traumatic brain injury: A double edged-sword. Current Opinion in Critical Care. 2002;**8**:101-105

[47] Salo M. Effect of anaesthesia and surgery on the immune response. Acta Anaesthesiologica Scandinavica. 1992;**36**:201-205

Chapter 7

Sedation in TBI Patients

Lorenzo Peluso, Berta Monleon Lopez and Rafael Badenes

Abstract

Sedation is an important topic in neurocritical patients. When compared with general intensive care unit and traumatic brain-injured patients, sedation has its therapeutic indications, such as management of intracranial pressure, treatment of status epilepticus, sedation for targeted temperature management patients and paroxysmal sympathetic activity. Nowadays, the assessment of sedation is done by neurological evaluation and new monitors based on electroencephalography signals that help the physician titrate the sedative agents. Therefore, the aim of this chapter is to discuss the main pharmacological properties of sedatives and analgesics, their proper indications related to pathophysiological issues and their titrations based on the abovementioned new technologies.

Keywords: TBI, sedation, sedative agent

1. Introduction

Traumatic brain injury is an acquired brain injury which occurs after a sudden trauma.

TBI is a major socioeconomic problem. It is an important cause of death and hospital admissions worldwide. The epidemiology in Europe is not well known, and more rigorous epidemiological studies are needed to fully quantify the effect of TBI society.

There are primary and secondary injuries. The primary injury is the trauma suffered by the patient itself, while the secondary injuries develop afterwards due to hypoxia, alterations in cerebral hemodynamic and metabolism and disruption of the blood brain barrier. Our aim is to avoid the secondary insults. Examples which can lead to worsen primary injury are convulsions, fever or intracranial hypertension.

TBI can be divided into different categories based on clinical examination or CT imaging. The most widely used is the Glasgow Coma Scale (GCS) based on neurological examination. Three categories can be found: mild, moderate, and severe. Other neurological scales used are based on time of loss of consciousness (LOC) (**Tables 1** and **2**) [1–3].

Many patients being admitted to the ICU are already under sedation due to neurological reasons. Nowadays, sedative agents are used either as a tool to apply other therapies (such as hypothermia) or as a treatment itself, for example, barbiturate coma for refractory hypertension.

Sedation and analgesia are practices that, all clinicians who provide care to patients affected by traumatic brain injury, have to face daily. These patients are usually excluded from randomized clinical trials, so the level of evidence in this setting is still low. The aims of sedation and analgesia can be divided into two main categories.

Firstly, general objectives are to ensure the patients' comfort, reduction of pain and agitation, improvement of patient-ventilator synchrony and facilitation of the nursing caring.

Parameter	Response	Score
Best eye-opening response	-Spontaneously	4
	-To verbal request	3
	-To pain	2
	-No response	1
Best verbal response	-Oriented and conversational	5
	-Disoriented and conversational	4
	-Inappropriate words	3
	-Incomprehensible sounds	2
	-No response	1
Best motor response	-Obesity request	6
	-Appropriate withdrawal	5
	-Flexion withdrawal	4
	-Flexion decorticate	3
	-Extension	2
	-No response	1

Table 1.
GCS classification

	GCS	LOC
Mild	14–15	0–30 min
Moderate	9–13	30 min–24 h
Severe	3–8	>24 h

Table 2.
TBI classification: GCS and LOC time.

Specific objectives focused on "neurotreatment" are the reduction of intracranial pressure (ICP), the management of status epilepticus (SE), the control of targeted temperature management (TTM), the management of paroxysmal sympathetic activity and the decrease of cerebral oxygen consumption [1, 2].

A variety of studies show the positive outcomes of an adequate sedation and analgesia in the general critical care patient as, for example, reduce time on the ventilator and decrease the length of stay in ICU and prevention of neurologic deterioration, amongst others.

The best way to assess these patients is with the physical examination, allowing a clinical monitoring and timely detection of warning neurological signs; thus, the removal of the sedative agent is required. However, this can lead to a cerebral and hemodynamic derangement when sedation is abruptly stopped [3]. Cerebral hypoperfusion and raised ICP might result in an imbalance of energy supply and demand, especially for the injured brain and, therefore, aggravate the risk for metabolic distress and brain tissue hypoxia. It might lead to significant ICP elevation and cerebral perfusion pressure (CPP) reduction, but it has been shown that, in patients with a stable ICP and CPP readings, the wake-up tests remain the gold standard for clinical monitoring and detection of neurological changes [4].

Available drugs used for sedation are analgesics and sedatives. Evidence shows that combining them both in order to achieve the optimal level of sedation leads to a reduction in the appearance of adverse effects.

Control patients' level of sedation plays an important role in what recently has been described as the "ABCDE bundle." An evidence-based clinical approach improves patients' outcome and recovery [5] such as duration of mechanical ventilation, brain dysfunction (i.e., delirium and coma), physical restraints, ICU readmission rates, and discharge disposition of ICU survivors.

In this chapter we will go over the basis of sedation in TBI patients, as well as the pharmacology of the different drugs used and the main indication for such patients.

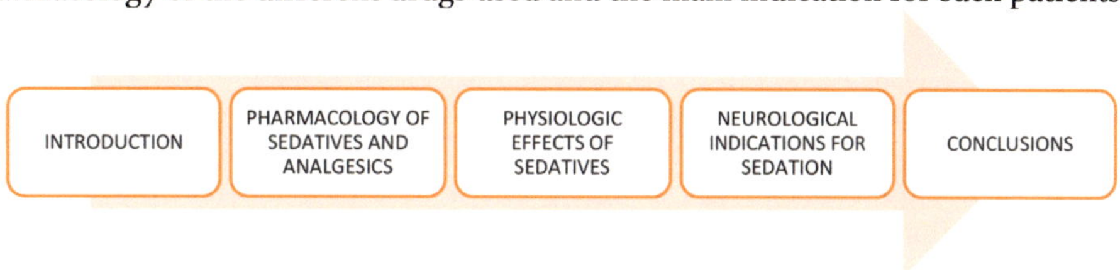

2. Pharmacology of sedatives and analgesics

The ideal sedative drug for a neurocritical patient should have different properties. It should have a rapid onset and recovery for a prompt neurologic evaluation, a predictable clearance independent of end-organ failure to avoid the accumulation of the drug, and it should be easily titrated. It has to reduce ICP by reducing cerebral blood flow (CBF) or cerebral vasoconstriction, however maintaining the coupling between cerebral blood flow and cerebral metabolic rate of oxygen consumption ($CMRO_2$). Cerebral autoregulation should be preserved as well as normal vascular reactivity to changes in $PaCO_2$. Finally, the hemodynamic depression should be minimal to avoid deleterious effects on brain circulation.

2.1 Propofol

Propofol is a central nervous system depressant which directly activates GABA receptors and inhibits the NMDA receptor modulating calcium influx through slow calcium ion channels. It has a rapid onset (1–2 min) and a dose-related hypnotic effect. Its rapid onset is due to its high lipophilic property and a large volume of distribution, leading to a rapid recovery too (10–15 min). These characteristics made propofol one of the best alternatives for sedation in neurocritical patients allowing us to do wake-up test daily for neurologic evaluation. Some studies show that in patients requiring >48 h of mechanical ventilation [6], sedation with propofol results in significantly fewer ventilator days than intermittent lorazepam when sedatives are interrupted daily. Propofol has no active metabolites and does not produce significant drug interactions. It reduces ICP, $CMRO_2$, CBF and cerebral electrical activity. CO_2 vascular reactivity and cerebral autoregulation are also preserved. On the other hand, it has no analgesic effect, and it raises tolerance and tachyphylaxis. Side effects of propofol are dose-dependent hypotension which can decrease cerebral perfusion pressure even if it induces a decrease in ICP [6] and dose-dependent respiratory depression. Thus, invasive blood pressure and maybe cardiac output monitoring may be necessary.

Hypertriglyceridemia may appear after high-rate infusions; clinicians should also be aware of the propofol infusion syndrome (PRIS) to detect it as soon as possible. PRIS manifests as metabolic acidosis, hyperkalemia, rhabdomyolysis, hypoxia and progressive myocardial failure [7–9].

2.2 Benzodiazepines

Benzodiazepines such as midazolam, lorazepam and diazepam are sedatives widely used in the ICU. They have anxiolytic, sedative and hypnotic properties. Midazolam is a GABA receptor agonist. Systemic effects of these drugs are anxiolysis, sedation, muscle relaxation, anterograde amnesia, respiratory depression and anticonvulsant activity. It decreases $CMRO_2$ and CBF and has a slight effect on lowering ICP too. As with propofol, vascular reactivity to CO_2 and cerebral autoregulation is preserved. Midazolam produces amnesia and has a rapid onset of action, and it produces less hemodynamic instability than propofol. However, they also produce tolerance and tachyphylaxis. Their metabolism is impaired when hepatic failure because of its oxidation via CYP450 enzyme system producing active metabolites excreted in the urine, leading to accumulation in renal dysfunction. It can prolong duration of mechanical ventilation, and the appearance of delirium in the ICU patients is increased. A continuous infusion of midazolam for more than 24 h will lose the rapid recovery properties due to the accumulation of active metabolites. Therefore, it is recommended only for short-term infusions. The Society of Critical Care Medicine consensus guidelines state that midazolam should be used only for short-term (<48 h) therapy [10]. High doses of benzodiazepines can cause respiratory depression and apnea, leading to an increase in ICP caused by hypercapnia. Benzodiazepines' reverser is flumazenil.

2.3 Opioids

Morphine, fentanyl and remifentanil are the most frequently used opioids in the ICU [11]. These drugs stimulate mu, kappa and delta receptors, distributed all along the central nervous system (CNS). They have a fast onset when given intravenous (iv), and they are more easily titrated. Morphine and meperidine are not the ideal sedative agent for ICU because their active metabolite can precipitate seizures [12]. Moreover, morphine has a long-lasting effect. Fentanyl with its high lipid solubility has a very rapid onset and a short duration of action when given as a bolus; however, the pharmacokinetics change when administered in perfusion. It may increase ICP and decrease CPP (decrease in MAP) transiently after a bolus. Remifentanil is more powerful than morphine, and it is metabolized directly in the plasma by nonspecific esterases, thus avoiding drug accumulation. Due to its very short duration of action, it requires a continuous perfusion [13–17]. This makes this drug very suitable for neurocritical patients because it facilitates frequent awakening for the neurologic evaluation [18]. Remifentanil is eliminated by the kidneys, and it does not have to be adjusted if kidney failure. On the other side, as they act as respiratory depressants, they may cause hypercapnia with consequent increase in ICP. They can induce histamine release, causing urticaria and flushing, somnolence respiratory depression, chest wall and other muscle rigidity, dysphoria or hallucinations, nausea and vomiting, gastrointestinal dysmotility and vasodilation with hypotension. The reverser is naloxone, which should be given slowly and be titrated.

In order to reduce and minimize the use of opioids, it is possible to add other categories of analgesics as gabapentin and/or acetaminophen [19].

2.4 Dexmedetomidine

Dexmedetomidine is an alpha-2 agonist which has been recently introduced into clinical practice. It has sedative, analgesic and anxiolytic properties, and it is widely starting to spread through the neurointensive care unit (NICU). It has a short-acting effect, and it does not accumulate, thus being very appropriate for frequently wake-up test for neurological evaluation. The respiratory depression is minimal, and it has been reported that it may reduce the incidence and severity of delirium. On the other side, it is a very expensive drug, and there have been reported cases of dose-dependent bradycardia, hypotension, arrhythmias and hyperglycemia. Deep sedation is not possible with this drug [20–24]. The pharmacokinetics is influenced by liver rather than renal function. Dexmedetomidine is metabolized in the liver by

CYP450 enzyme system, and there are no active or toxic metabolites. Sedation with volunteers showed a decrease in regional and global cerebral blood flow, but the ratio with $CMRO_2$ and flow metabolism coupling is maintained [25]. The neuroprotective effect in animal studies has also been studied, and they showed a preconditioning effect and attenuation of ischemia-reperfusion injury [26].

2.5 Barbiturates

Nowadays, these drugs are used only for a specific goal. They are a GABA receptor agonist leading to a decrease in ICP and CBF that is proportional to the decrease in $CMRO_2$ (up to 60%) during burst suppression. Barbiturates have been associated with a high incidence of systemic complications, such as hemodynamic instability and immune suppression with an increased risk of infections, such as pneumonia. Indication for barbiturates is limited to refractory intracranial hypertension and refractory status epilepticus [27]. They accumulate in the tissues after long-term infusions leading to slow recovery from sedation.

2.6 Ketamine

Ketamine is an NMDA receptor antagonist with a relatively good hemodynamic stability. It has a fast onset and a short action. Sedation, analgesia and anesthesia can be induced with this drug, and it does not depress the respiratory system. Potential side effects of ketamine are increase of $CMRO_2$, CBF and ICP (due to an increase in cerebral blood volume). However, some reports have shown to decrease CBF and ICP in head trauma patients sedated using both ketamine and propofol or with a $PaCO_2$ maintained constant [28], and in an experimental setting ketamine even had neuroprotective properties [29]. Main advantages of using ketamine are the hemodynamic stability as well as CPP and the opportunity to reduce the excessive use of some sedative drugs as it reinforces them.

In a recent study, the use of ketamine was associated with a lower incidence of cortical spreading depolarization (CSD) when compared with propofol, midazolam and opioids [30].

2.7 Inhalation sedatives

Inhalative sedation in the ICU is starting to spread all over Europe and has been recommended as an alternative in a German consensus guideline [31]. However, it has historically been considered unsafe in the NICU around the world. Isoflurane, sevoflurane, and desflurane have shown some benefits compared with intravenous sedation. They have a low metabolism and, due to their low solubility, are eliminated quickly and offer shorter and more predictable wake-up times than intravenous agents. They give also a better hemodynamic stability. Some volatile anesthetics abolish cerebral autoregulation at high doses; it has been reported that with sevoflurane at MAC 1.0, the autoregulation of cerebral blood flow remained intact, but it was impaired at MAC 2.0. They have also a dose-dependent neuroprotective effect; sevoflurane at MAC 0.5 does not have this effect [32].

In a prospective study, it was seen that sufficient sedation levels without clinically relevant ICP increases were achieved in 68% of the patients. However, MAP had to be maintained actively to preserve the CPP. Therefore, it was concluded that the neuroprotective effect did not outweigh the risk of adverse events, and sedation with this agent should not be carry out in these patients [33].

A summary table can be found at the end of the chapter.

	Mechanism of action	Rapid onset	Fast recovery	Metabolism	IV Bolus dose	Continuous IV infusion	ICP reduction	CBF reduction	$CMRO_2$ reduction	Map reduction	Main advantages	Main disadvantages	Adverse effects
Propofol	GABA R agonist	+++	+++	Hepatic	1.5–2.5 mg/kg	5–200 mg/kg/min	↓↓	↓↓	↓↓	↓↓	Clearance independent of renal or hepatic function. Rapid onset and fast recovery	No analgesia. Tolerance and tachyphylaxis. Increases triglycerides.	PRIS. Hypotension
Midazolam	GABA R agonist	+++	++	Hepatic	0.02–0.08 mg/kg	0.04–0.3 mg/kg/h	↓	↓↓	↓	↓	Amnesia. Rapid onset	Tolerance. Tachyphylaxis. Accumulates in renal dysfunction. Active metabolites	Hypotension. Apnea. Delirium
Morphine	MU-R agonist	+	+	Hepatic	0.8–10 mg/h	Max 80 mg/h	↓/=	=	↓	↓/=	Less peripheric accumulation than fentanyl. Analgesia	Hypotension	Apnea. Hypotension. Pruritus. Nausea. Active metabolite can produce seizures. Muscle rigidity
Fentanyl	MU-R agonist	+++	++	Hepatic	25–125 mg	10–100 mg/h	↓/=	=	↓	↓	More potent analgesic than morphine	Accumulation with hepatic impairment. Apnea	Pruritus. Nausea. Muscle rigidity.
Remifentanil	MU-R agonist	+++	+++	Plasmatic esterases		0.05–0.25 mg/kg/min	↓/=	=	↓	↓	500× more potent than morphine		Hyperalgesia after infusion. CV depressant.
Dexdor	ALPHA 2 agonist	++	++	Hepatic	Not recommended	0.2–1.4 mg/kg/h	↓/=	↓	↓	↓	Sedative, anxiolytic, analgesic. Minimal respiratory depression. Reduces delirium	Limited experience in ABI.	Arrhythmias. Hypotension. Bradicardia.
Thiopental	GABA R agonist	+++	+	Hepatic	2–5 mg/kg	1–5 mg/kg/h	↓↓	↓↓	↓↓	↓↓	Second-line treatment for refractory intracraneal hypertension	Accumulates in peripheral tissue. Adjust dose in renal failure.	HD instability. Immunosuppression.

	Mechanism of action	Rapid onset	Fast recovery	Metabolism	IV Bolus dose	Continuous IV infusion	ICP reduction	CBF reduction	$CMRO_2$ reduction	Map reduction	Main advantages	Main disadvantages	Adverse effects
Ketamine	NMDA R agonist	+++	+++	Liver	1–4 mg/kg	(0.5–2 mg/kg)	↑/=	↓	↓	↑/=	Sedation, anesthesia, analgesia. No respiratory depression. HD stability.	Increases secretions.	Hallucinations. Nystagmus. Increases IOP, IAP
Sevorane	Not clear. GABA R agonist + glutamate receptor agonist	+++	++	5% Hepatic. 95% inhalatory pathway	2% MAC	0.5–3% of sevorane in	May increase after increase in CBF	↑	↓	↓	Fast elimination. Increases CBF in cerebral ischemia.	Hypotension. MAC 2 autoregulation impairs.	Toxic metabolite (compound A). Malignant hyperthermia

3. Physiologic effects of sedatives on cerebral blood flow and cerebral metabolic rate of oxygen consumption

Sedation is one of the pillars in the management of patients with TBI. It is a treatment itself when used to prevent the secondary insult, and it allows other measures to be implemented which could not be applied otherwise, such as hypothermia.

The physiologic effects of sedatives are different, and they can be divided into effects on CBF and $CMRO_2$.

3.1 Effects on cerebral blood flow (CBF)

One of the main goals when treating these patients is to maintain a sufficient cerebral blood flow. Therefore, our drugs should have little or no effect on this matter.

The effects of intravenous sedatives on CBF have been investigated for diazepam, midazolam and propofol. All these iv agents cause a dose-dependent decrease in $CMRO_2$ and CBF. CBF reduction is an adaptative phenomenon to minimize brain metabolism. They usually have a systemic effect decreasing mean arterial pressure (MAP), inducing myocardial depression and peripheral vasodilation. Therefore, in patients with impaired autoregulation, such as those with TBI, decreasing the MAP can lead to a critical lowering in cerebral perfusion pressure and oxygen delivery to the brain. This can lead or worsen the secondary brain insult (ischemia/hypoxia) [34, 35]. If autoregulation is intact, this reduction on MAP will produce reflex cerebral vasodilation and may lead to an increase in intracranial pressure [36]. The hemodynamic effects are usually dose dependent, so it is important to assess the preload status of the patient in order to predict the hemodynamic response to the sedative agent, particularly in those with previous cardiac dysfunction.

3.2 Effects on the cerebral metabolic rate of oxygen consumption ($CMRO_2$)

The $CMRO_2$ and CBF are nicely connected. In TBI patients, our target is to maintain an adequate oxygen availability and energy balance; thus, we aim to increase oxygen delivery by optimizing cerebral and systemic hemodynamic, as well as attenuating metabolic demands [2, 37, 38].

Patients in coma or suffering from secondary brain insults have their cerebral metabolism decreased globally by one-third to one-half of normal levels.

Sedative agents act by reducing CMRO2, improving cerebral tolerance to ischemia and limiting the supply/demand mismatch in conditions of impaired autoregulation [34, 35]. Beyond the level of isoelectric EEG, no further suppression of cerebral oxygen consumption can take place; a minimal oxygen consumption is, indeed, due to cells' homeostasis.

4. Neurological indications for sedation

Continuous infusion of sedative agents is contemplated during the first 48 h, in order to prevent secondary brain injury by decreasing oxygen consumption, as well as to reduce pain, anxiety and agitation to tolerate mechanical ventilation.

Apart from the general indications due to patient's agitation and pain control, there are specific situations in these patients that require sedation as therapy.

4.1 Control of intracranial pressure (ICP)

The effect of sedatives on ICP is due mainly to reduction in $CMRO_2$ that leads to a decrease in cerebral blood flow. This effect can be seen as a decrease in cerebral blood volume that leads to a decrease in ICP. As well, sedation reduces pain and agitation and improves the tolerance to the endotracheal tube. These effects lead to a decrease of sympathetic activity with a reduction of arterial pressure and less ventilation asynchronies leading to a decrease of jugular venous resistance and a better venous outflow.

Sedation is a first-line therapy that should be integrated with other specific interventions as hyperventilation, osmotic agents and head-of-bed elevation. Bolus of opioids needs caution for the transient decrease in mean arterial pressure and increase in ICP due to autoregulatory cerebral vasodilation [36]. When compared with opioids, propofol showed an association with a lower ICP and less ICP treatments in patients with severe traumatic brain injury (TBI) [6].

4.2 Targeted temperature management (TTM)

The effects of hypothermia on the brain are multiple. First, the cerebral metabolic rate decreases leading to a decrease in CBF and, consequently, a reduction of cerebral volume. Moreover, cooling procedures suppress many of the pathways that lead to cell death, including apoptotic mechanisms (programmed cell death).

Sedation is recommended during TTM to prevent shivering, to reduce the stress response and to allow the patient-ventilator synchrony. To avoid shivering a lot of drugs are available, but they could engender side effects. One of the most used drugs is propofol that has a dose-dependent antishivering effect.

An excess in sedation can lead to an increase of mechanical ventilation time and a delay in neurological response [39].

4.3 Treatment of status epilepticus (SE)

Status epilepticus is a quite common neurologic condition with an overall incidence of 41–61 cases per 100,000 patients/year [40].

The emergency therapy consists in benzodiazepines for the emergency, followed by one or more anti-epileptic drugs (AED). When both categories fail, it is necessary to begin a deep sedation with anesthetic agents for at least 24 h of effectiveness [41].

Different studies showed and reported the effectiveness of propofol or midazolam as therapy for refractory SE.

The traditional barbiturate (phenobarbital), due to its side effects, is being replaced by the newest propofol and midazolam.

4.4 Paroxysmal sympathetic activity

This syndrome has been recognized in a subgroup of survivors of severe acquired brain injury, characterized by simultaneous, paroxysmal transient increases in sympathetic (elevated heart rate, blood pressure, respiratory rate, temperature, sweating) and motor (posturing) activity. This syndrome has been observed for the last 60 years. It affects 8–10% of patients suffering from acute brain injury, and it is associated with greater morbidity, higher healthcare costs, longer hospitalization and poorer outcomes. However, it is a potentially treatable contributor to secondary brain injury. In patients surviving traumatic brain injury, it has been associated with severe anoxia, subarachnoid and intracerebral hemorrhage and hydrocephalus. There are many theories dealing with the pathophysiology of this entity. Disconnection of the inhibitory efferent pathways (malfunctioning pathways) from cortical areas of the brain is one of the possible theories. It is also thought that alterations in the excitatory nucleus of the brainstem can cause this syndrome; excitatory centers are then upregulated, increasing sympathetic activity. There is no accepted treatment for this entity. The objective is to mitigate signs and symptoms to avoid the adverse effects such as dehydration, muscle wasting or delayed recovery. Dopaminergic agents have shown to decrease body temperature and sweating. Alpha agonists can decrease heart rate and blood pressure. When medication fails, the use of hyperbaric oxygen therapy (HBOT) to control autonomic discharges and posturing in the subacute TBI phase has been reported. In this condition, sedation should be considered to reduce sympathetic activation [42].

5. Monitoring sedation in the neuro-ICU

Monitoring the depth of sedation is essential in the management of the patient in the ICU, and it influences their outcomes. Oversedation increases the risk of infections by delaying weaning from mechanical ventilation and increases length of stay and, thus, costs. On the other side, undersedation can cause agitation and anxiety of the patient, increase the risk of self-extubating and develop asynchronies between the patient and the ventilator. In NICU patients, assessing routine level of sedation is really important both for the daily wake-up tests that should be done for neurologic evaluation and, in comatose patients, to avoid oversedation.

There are various scales available for ICU patients. The Ramsay Sedation Scale evaluates consciousness, while the Richmond Agitation-Sedation Scale (RASS) examines cognition. The Motor Activity Assessment Scale (MAAS) and the Sedation-Agitation Scale (SAS) monitor sedation and arousal. Both RASS and SAS are reasonable to use in TBI patients [43]. Moreover, RASS is usually integrated with a delirium assessment performed with Confusion Assessment Method for the ICU (CAM-ICU). However, in deeply sedated patients and with muscular blockade, these scales become useless. EEG monitoring has therefore become a very investigated topic to titrate sedation in these patients. Simplified EEG tools like BIS, based on Fourier transform, have shown significant correlation with RASS and SAS in ABI [44]. However, BIS was developed to monitor sedation in the operating room (OR) setting in patients with no acute brain injury (ABI) due to the possible changes in EEG because of the brain lesion; it is often used in the ICU setting.

The possible confounders of such method are shivering, temperature fluctuation, increased muscle tone, grimacing and catecholamine levels. To assess the adequacy of pain relief, it is useful to assess autonomic signs of activation such as tachycardia, hypertension, ICP increase and diaphoresis.

6. Conclusions

Sedation and analgesia are widely used in NICU and all clinicians who provide care to neuropatients' face daily with such practice. The indication for sedation in NICU could be general or properly neurologic that is considered as a therapy in the acute brain injury patient. Sedation, indeed, allows a better control of cerebral hemodynamic and is part of control of intracranial pressure.

The knowledge of basic principles of pharmacology, neurophysiology, and neuropathology remains, therefore, essential to manage such kind of therapy.

Propofol and midazolam seem to be the most used drugs in such patient due to their security profile; ketamine appears to be interesting for its neuroprotective role.

To target sedation properly, it is possible to use different approaches; the use of score (RASS, SAS) in the awake patient remains a good tool that can be integrated in comatose patient, knowing their limits, with the newest EEG-derived methods.

Conflict of interest

We declare no conflict of interest.

Author details

Lorenzo Peluso[1], Berta Monleon Lopez[2] and Rafael Badenes[2]*

1 Department of Intensive Care Hôpital Erasme, Brussels, Belgium

2 Department of Anesthesiology and Surgical-Trauma Intensive Care, Hospital Clìnico Universitario, Valencia, Spain

*Address all correspondence to: rafaelbadenes@gmail.com

References

[1] Kress JP, Pohlman AS, O'Connor MF, Hall JB. Daily interruption of sedative infusions in critically ill patients undergoing mechanical ventilation. The New England Journal of Medicine. 2000;**342**:1471-1477

[2] A Villa F, Citerio G. Sedation and analgesia in neurointensive care. In: Textbook of Neurointensive Care. 2nd ed. London: Springer; 2013. pp. 281-292

[3] Oddo M, Crippa IA, Mehta S, Menon D, Payen JF, Taccone FS, et al. Optimizing sedation in patients with acute brain injury. Critical Care. 2016; **20**(1):128

[4] Marklund N. The neurological wake-up test-A role in neurocritical care monitoring of traumatic brain injury patients? Frontiers in Neurology. 2017;**8**: 540

[5] Morandi A, Brummel NE, Ely EW. Sedation, delirium and mechanical ventilation: The "ABCDE" approach. Current Opinion in Critical Care. 2011; **17**(1):43-49

[6] Kelly DF, Goodale DB, Williams J, et al. Propofol in the treatment of moderate and severe head injury: A randomized, prospective, double-blinded pilot trial. Journal of Neurosurgery. 1999;**90**:1042-1052

[7] Cannon ML, Glazier SS, Bauman LA. Metabolic acidosis, rhabdomyolysis, and cardiovascular collapse after prolonged propofol infusion. Journal of Neurosurgery. 2001;**95**:1053-1056

[8] Kelly DF. Propofol-infusion syndrome. Journal of Neurosurgery. 2001;**95**:925-926

[9] Laham J. Propofol: Risk vs. benefit. Clinical Pediatrics (Phila). 2002; **41**(1):5-7

[10] Devlin JW, Skrobik Y, Gélinas C, et al. Clinical practice guidelines for the prevention and management of Pain, agitation/sedation, delirium, immobility, and sleep disruption in adult patients in the ICU. Critical Care Medicine. 2018;**46**:e825-e873

[11] Mehta S, Burry L, Fischer S, et al. Canadian survey of the use of sedatives, analgesics, and neuromuscular blocking agents in critically ill patients. Critical Care Medicine. 2006;**34**(2):374-380

[12] Armstrong PJ, Bersten A. Normeperidine toxicity. Anesthesia and Analgesia. 1986;**65**(5):536-538

[13] Pitsiu M, Wilmer A, Bodenham A, et al. Pharmacokinetics of remifentanil and its major metabolite, remifentanil acid, in ICU patients with renal impairment. British Journal of Anaesthesia. 2004;**92**:493-503

[14] Dumont L, Picard V, Marti RA, et al. Use of remifentanil in a patient with chronic hepatic failure. British Journal of Anaesthesia. 1998;**81**:265-267

[15] Egan TD, Lemmens HJ, Fiset P, et al. The pharmacokinetics of the new short-acting opioid remifentanil (GI87084B) in healthy adult male volunteers. Anesthesiology. 1993;**79**(5):881-892

[16] Delvaux B, Ryckwaert Y, Van Boven M, et al. Remifentanil in the intensive care unit: Tolerance and acute withdrawal syndrome after prolonged sedation. Anesthesiology. 2005;**102**(6): 1281-1282

[17] Karabinis A, Mandragos K, Stergiopoulos S, et al. Safety and efficacy of analgesia-based sedation with remifentanil versus standard hypnotic-based regimens in intensive care unit patients with brain injuries: A randomised, controlled trial

[ISRCTN50308308]. Critical Care. 2004;**8**(4):R268-R280

[18] Belleville JP. Effects of intravenous dexmedetomidine in humans: Part I: Sedation, ventilation, and metabolic rate. Anesthesiology. 1992;**77**:1125-1133

[19] Barr J, Fraser GL, Puntillo K, et al. Clinical practice guidelines for the management of pain agitation and delirium in adult patients in the intensive care unit. Critical Care Medicine. 2013;**41**(263):306

[20] Bloor BC, Ward DS, Belleville JP, et al. Effects of intravenous dexmedetomidine in humans: Part II: Hemodynamic changes. Anesthesiology. 1992;**77**:1134-1142

[21] Talke P, Richardson CA, Scheinin M, et al. Postoperative pharmacokinetics and sympatholytic effects of dexmedetomidine. Anesthesia and Analgesia. 1997;**85**:1136-1142

[22] Triltsch AE, Welte M, von Homeyer P, et al. Bispectral index—Guided sedation with dexmedetomidine in intensive care: A prospective, randomized, double blind, placebo-controlled phase II study. Critical Care Medicine. 2002;**30**:1007-1014

[23] Venn RM, Bryant A, Hall GM, et al. Effects of dexmedetomidine on adrenocortical function, and the cardiovascular, endocrine and inflammatory responses in postoperative patients needing sedation in the intensive care unit. British Journal of Anaesthesia. 2001;**86**:650-656

[24] Drummond JC, Dao AV, Roth DM, et al. Effect of dexmedetomidine on cerebral blood flow velocity, cerebral metabolic rate, and carbon dioxide response in normal humans. Anesthesiology. 2008;**108**:225-232

[25] Dahmani S, Rouelle D, Gressens P, et al. Effects of dexmedetomidine on hippocampal focal adhesion kinase tyrosine phosphorylation in physiologic and ischemic conditions. Anesthesiology. 2005;**103**:969-977

[26] Bratton SL, Chestnut RM, Ghajar J, et al. Guidelines for the m anagement of severe traumatic brain injury XI. Anesthetics, analgesics, and sedatives. Journal of Neurotrauma. 2007;**24** (Supp. 1):S71-S76

[27] Albanèse J, Arnaud S, Rey M, et al. Ketamine decreases intracranial pressure and electroencephalographic activity in traumatic brain injury patients during propofol sedation. Anesthesiology. 1997;**87**(6):1328-1334

[28] Shapira Y, Lam AM, Eng CC, et al. Therapeutic time window and dose response of the beneficial effects of ketamine in experimental head injury. Stroke. 1994;**25**:1637-1643

[29] Martin J et al. Evidence and consensus-based German guidelines for the management of analgesia, sedation and delirium in intensive care-short version. German Medical Science. 2010; **8**:Doc02

[30] Hertle DN, Dreier JP, Woitzik J, et al. Effect of analgesics and sedatives on the occurrence of spreading depolarizations accompanying acute brain injury. Brain. 2012;**135**(Pt 8): 2390-2398

[31] Xie Z et al. The inhalation anesthetic isoflurane induces a vicious cycle of apoptosis and amyloid beta-protein accumulation. The Journal of Neuroscience. 2007;**27**:1247-1254

[32] Purruker JC, Renzland J, Uhlmann L. Volatile sedation with sevoflurane in intensive care patients with acute stroke or subarachnoid haemorrhage using AnaConDa®: An observational study. British Journal of Anaesthesia. 2015;**114**: 934-943

[33] Riker RR, Fugate JE, et al. Clinical monitoring scales in acute brain injury: Assessment of coma, pain, agitation, and delirium. Neurocritical Care. 2014; **21**(Supp. 2):S27-S37

[34] Stephan H, Sonntag H, Schenk HD, Kohlhausen S. Effect of Disoprivan (propofol) on the circulation and oxygen consumption of the brain and CO_2 reactivity of brain vessels in the human. Anaesthesist. 1987;**36**(2):60-65

[35] Van Hemelrijck J, Fitch W, Mattheussen M, Van Aken H, Plets C, Lauwers T. Effect of propofol on cerebral circulation and autoregulation in the baboon. Anesthesia and Analgesia. 1990;**71**:49-54

[36] Albanese J, Viviand X, Potie F, Rey M, Alliez B, Martin C. Sufentanil, fentanyl, and alfentanil in head trauma patients: A study on cerebral hemodynamics. Critical Care Medicine. 1999;**27**:407-411

[37] Kress JP, Pohlman AS, Hall JB. Sedation and analgesia in the intensive care unit. American Journal of Respiratory and Critical Care Medicine. 2002;**166**:1024-1028

[38] Oddo M, Steiner LA. Sedation and analgesia in the neurocritical care unit. In: Smith M, Kofke WA, Citerio G, editors. Oxford Textbook of Neurocritical Care. Oxford: Oxford University Press; 2016

[39] Samaniego EA, Mlynash M, Caulfield AF, et al. Sedation confounds outcome prediction in cardiac arrest survivors treated with hypothermia. Neurocritical Care. 2011;**15**:113-119

[40] De Lorenzo RJ, Hauser WA, Towne AR, et al. A prospective, population-based epidemiologic study of status epilepticus in Richmond, Virginia. Neurology. 1996;**46**(4):1029-1035

[41] Rossetti AO, Bleck TP. What's new in status epilepticus? Intensive Care Medicine. 2014;**40**:1359-1362

[42] Perkes I, Baguley IJ, Nott MT, et al. A review of paroxysmal sympathetic hyperactivity after acquired brain injury. Annals of Neurology. 2010;**68**: 126-135

[43] Deogaonkar A, Gupta R, DeGeorgia M, Sabharwal V, Gopakumaran B, Schubert A, et al. Bispectral index monitoring correlates with sedation scales in brain-injured patients. Critical Care Medicine. 2004;**32**:2403-2406

[44] Pandharipande P, Shintani A, Peterson J, et al. Lorazepam is an independent risk factor for transitioning to delirium in intensive care unit patients. Anesthesiology. 2006;**104**: 21-26